Stay Cool Through Menopause

Answers To Your Most-Asked Questions

Melvin Frisch, M.D.

THE BODY PRESS/PERIGEE

Notice: The information in this book is true and complete to the best of our knowledge. The book is intended only as a guide. It is not intended as a replacement for sound medical advice from a doctor. Only a doctor can include the variables of an individual's age and medical history needed for wise medical advice. Final decision about any medical action must be made by the individual and her doctor. All recommendations herein are made without guarantees on the part of the author or the publisher. The author and publisher disclaim all liability in connection with the use of this information.

The Body Press/Perigee Books
are published by
The Putnam Publishing Group
200 Madison Avenue
New York, NY 10016

Library of Congress Cataloging-in-Publication Data

Frisch, Melvin J., date.
  Stay cool through menopause : answers to your most-asked questions / Melvin Frisch.
     p.   cm.
  Includes bibliographical references and index.
  ISBN 0-399-51818-5
  1. Menopause—Miscellanea.   I. Title
RG186.F75   1993   92-41801 CIP
612.6'5—dc20

Cover design by Judith Kazdym Leeds
Printed in the United States of America
     2   3   4   5   6   7   8   9   10

Acknowledgments

I would like to give special thanks to my wife, Patti, who helped me with the manuscript by making sure the medical terminology was easy to understand, and to her friends and her book club, who gave me the initial ideas for the book. I also would like to thank my patients, who, over the last several years, have supplied many of the questions answered here.

Table of Contents

Prologue

In 1987, when I began working on the first edition of this book, there was very little interest in and very few books about menopause. Now, several years later, menopause appears to have made it "out of the closet." Hardly a day goes by without a newspaper or magazine story on hormone therapy or the emotional and medical aspects of menopause.

Stay Cool Through Menopause is unique among books about menopause in that it in effect gives the reader a comprehensive consultation with a physician about all aspects of the subject. It answers specific questions women have about the symptoms and treatment of menopause. The book is written from the perspective of a physician who deals with menopause on a daily basis in his office. The majority of my professional medical practice is devoted to menopause, whether in treating patients or teaching medical students and physicians specializing in obstetrics and gynecology.

In the 1960s several medical reports were published claiming that women could use estrogen replacement therapy during and after menopause and remain young and vigorous, with wrinkle-free skin. As a result, many women began taking estrogen. In 1976 a report in *The New England Journal of Medicine* showed a link between estrogen and endometrial cancer. This study, as well as others, frightened both physicians and their patients away from estrogen therapy, and its use in treating the postmenopausal symptoms of hot flashes, irregular periods, and vaginal dryness became very unpopular.

Today, approximately forty million women in the United States are past menopause, representing an increase of thir-

Chart P-1

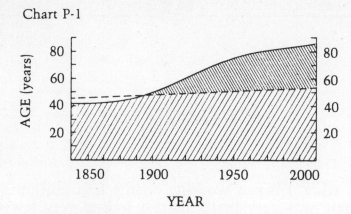

Relationship between female life expectancy and
age at the time of menopause showing the
increasing number of years women are living after
menopause.

teen million over the last decade or two. The average life
expectancy for a woman is eighty years, so she can expect
to live more than one-third of her life after menopause. (See
chart P-1.) This increase in the number of women living in
their postmenopausal years has renewed interest in allevi-
ating symptoms of menopause and preventing osteoporosis
and cardiovascular disease often prevalent during this time.
Attention has once again turned to estrogen replacement
therapy. Medical researchers feel that by combining estrogen
with the other female hormone progesterone, they have
found ways of prescribing hormones that are much safer and
have fewer side effects.

The menopausal years are characterized by a combination
of hormonal, physical, and psychological changes due to the
combined effects of estrogen deficiency and the natural aging process. It is often difficult to tell which symptoms may
be attributed to a lack of estrogen and which are actually

due to natural aging. Can such symptoms as inability to sleep and wrinkled skin previously attributed to the natural aging process, actually be caused by estrogen deficiency? Information in this book will answer this question and many others.

Women vary greatly in the amount of estrogen they produce around the time of menopause. The intensity of their symptoms also varies greatly and is correlated with changing estrogen levels. Many women continue to produce estrogen from sources other than their ovaries, *so it is important that women be evaluated and treated on an individual basis.*

In this book I wish to clarify many of the myths that have been associated with menopause and give a better understanding of what women may expect during the menopausal years. By reading the questions and answers here, you may be able to have an intelligent discussion with your doctor about the symptoms of and treatment for menopause. You will be making decisions about your health care that will affect you for the next thirty years, and I hope the information here will help you make those decisions that mean a happier, healthier life.

Melvin J. Frisch, M.D.

1

What Is Menopause?

As you approach your mid- to late-forties, you may begin to experience symptoms which can appear unusual and occasionally frightening. Although these symptoms may not be an immediate threat to your health, they can be troubling and may affect your well-being in the ensuing years. During the next twenty years your body will undergo many changes, some rather obvious, others so subtle you may be unaware of them. Most women of previous generations simply did not discuss menstrual abnormalities, hot flashes, night sweats, restless nights and other menopausal symptoms. This book was written to answer all your questions about the changes that your body undergoes during menopause, why those changes occur, the symptoms that can result, and what can be done to alleviate your discomfort.

What is menopause?

Menopause is the permanent cessation of menstruation. It can occur as early as age 35 or as late as age 55. Although we refer to the years before and after the last menstrual period as the menopausal years, in strict medical terminology, the word menopause means the last menstrual period. It is only one event in the *climateric,* a period of biological change in all body tissue and systems that occurs in both sexes between the ages of 40 and 60.

What is the climacteric?

The climacteric is that time in your life when your body undergoes a number of hormonal changes. In women, the climacteric is also referred to as the menopausal years. It is during this time that the ovaries stop producing estrogen and progesterone on a predictable basis and a woman's child-bearing years come to an end. It is a change from the reproductive to the nonreproductive years in a woman's life cycle.

What is the perimenopause?

The perimenopause are the years just before and after your last menstrual period. During this time your menses become irregular and sporadic until they ultimately cease. Physicians commonly refer to irregular and heavy menstrual bleeding that often occurs at this age as *perimenopausal bleeding*.

What causes menopause?

Menopause is caused by the gradual decrease of estrogen production by the ovaries, It is sometimes referred to as *ovarian failure* (the failure of the ovaries to produce estrogen). The causes of menopause are explained fully in the next chapter.

What is estrogen?

Estrogen is a group of related hormones that are produced primarily by the ovaries. Estrogen is responsible for sexual development of the female, such as breast development and menstruation. Many organs in your body need estrogen to function normally. The gradual decrease in the production of estrogen causes the onset of menopause.

MENOPAUSAL SYMPTOMS

What symptoms and concerns might I have during the menopausal years?

The major symptoms and concerns of women during the menopausal years include:

- irregular, heavy menstrual bleeding
- hot flashes, night sweats, and sleepless nights
- vaginal dryness with painful intercourse
- recurrent vaginal and bladder infections
- sleep disturbances, emotional instability, and anxiety
- wrinkled skin
- osteoporosis
- cardiovascular disease (heart attacks, stroke, and hypertension)
- breast disease
- other disorders of the reproductive organs, such as uterine fibroids and ovarian cysts

Do the symptoms occur in a predictable time sequence?

Although the age at which menopause occurs varies from woman to woman, the sequence of the symptoms is somewhat predictable. The following chart gives general guidelines for what to expect, assuming menopause occurs at age 50. If menopause begins earlier, say at age 40, each of the symptoms listed below would occur approximately ten years earlier. If, on the other hand, you continue to menstruate until you're 60, your symptoms will be delayed for an additional ten years.

AGE	SYMPTOMS
40–50	Irregular, heavy menstrual periods
48	Hot flashes and flushes
50	Menopause (the last menstrual period)
52	Hot flashes and flushes
54	Vaginal dryness with painful intercourse
56	Urinary and bladder symptoms
58	Cardiovascular disease including heart attacks
58	Osteoporosis

Does everyone have symptoms going through menopause?

No, some women just stop having their periods and have no further symptoms. Most women, however, will have some indication of decreased ovarian function, such as an occasional hot flash or irregular menstrual periods, but nothing serious enough to warrant seeking medical attention.

Generally, what are the most frequent complaints at the time of menopause?

The two most common complaints are hot flashes and vaginal dryness. Hot flashes may occur several years prior to the last menstrual period and can last for several years afterward. Some women may experience hot flashes while still having regular menstrual cycles.

What determines who has symptoms during menopause?

Doctors don't know why some women develop symptoms and others do not. Some women suffer a great deal of discomfort with hot flashes or vaginal dryness while others who appear to have the same body build and presumedly produce the same amount of estrogen, may not be affected at all. Every woman is different, so each symptom should be dealt with on an individual basis.

Chart 1-1

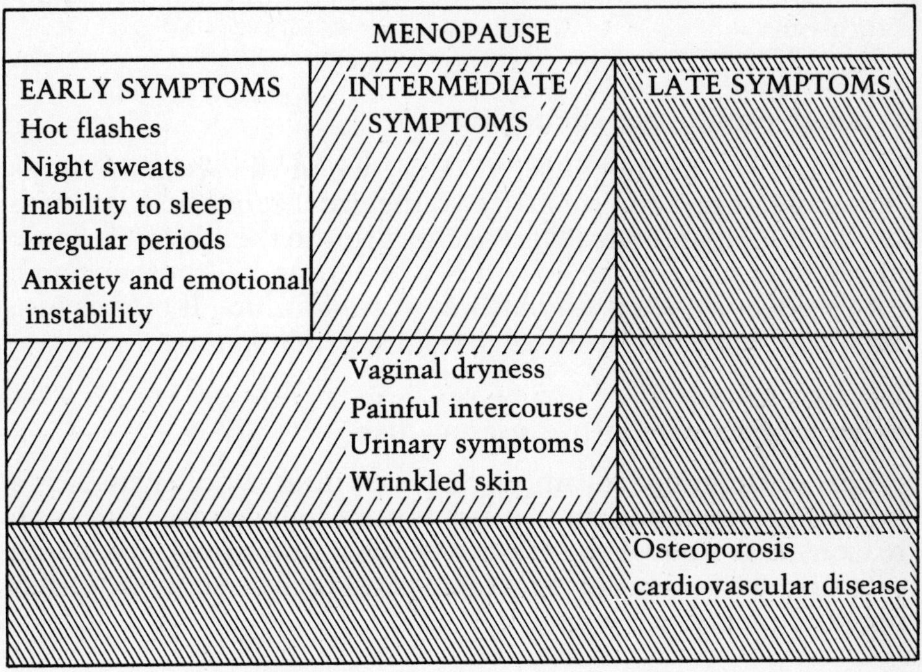

MENOPAUSE		
EARLY SYMPTOMS Hot flashes Night sweats Inability to sleep Irregular periods Anxiety and emotional instability	INTERMEDIATE SYMPTOMS	LATE SYMPTOMS
	Vaginal dryness Painful intercourse Urinary symptoms Wrinkled skin	
		Osteoporosis cardiovascular disease

Signs and symptoms of menopause.

THE TIMING OF YOUR MENOPAUSE

What is the average age for menopause?

Fifty is the average age at which a woman stops having her menstrual periods, but the onset of menopause usually occurs between the ages of 45 and 55. Approximately 8% of all women go through a natural menopause before the age of 40. A smaller percentage will continue to menstruate regularly into their late 50's, and even a few, into their early 60's.

How will I know when I have my last menstrual period?

The menopause or last menstrual period is always a retrospective event; you really won't know you've had your last menstrual period until you go twelve months without another one.

What is premature menopause?

Premature menopause occurs when a woman stops menstruating at an unusually young age. Menopause is usually considered premature if it occurs prior to the age of 45. Some physicians use the age of 40 as a benchmark. Another name for this occurrence is *premature ovarian failure*. If menopause occurs after age 55, it is called *delayed menopause*.

What causes premature menopause?

One of the most common, but least understood, causes is a hereditary predisposition to premature menopause. For some reason, a woman inherits fewer eggs and stops producing estrogen at an earlier age than most other women. Other possible factors include:

- **severe infections that destroy the ovarian tissue**
- **surgical removal of the ovaries**
- **previous irradiation or chemotherapy for cancer**
- **an autoimmune disease through which a woman's immune system attacks and destroys her own ovarian tissue**

What factors may influence the timing of the onset of my menopause?

Social habits, such as smoking, alcohol consumption, the altitude at which you live, your socioeconomic conditions, and your body composition, all influence when you will undergo menopause. Some of these factors have more of an impact than others.

Does smoking cause an early menopause?

It has been established that a woman who smokes more than half a pack a day undergoes menopause five to ten years earlier than other members in her family, all other factors being equal. Smoking also increases the risk of developing one of the more serious consequences of early menopause— osteoporosis. Smoking has a twofold effect on osteoporosis: it reduces the thickness of bone and it can cause an earlier menopause that predisposes a woman to osteoporosis.

Is there any correlation between alcohol consumption and early menopause?

There is evidence that women who drink heavily go through menopause at an earlier age than women who do not.

What effect does altitude have on menopause?

Studies have confirmed that women who live at higher elevations experience an earlier onset of menopause (by several years) than women in similar socioeconomic groups who live at lower altitudes.

Do socioeconomic factors influence menopause?

No one knows why women of higher socioeconomic status usually undergo a later menopause. Researchers suggest that education, nutrition, and a woman's general health status correlate with socioeconomic status to cause the later menopause. Factors such as family and working status, as well as stress levels, all may influence some of the psychological symptoms experienced at this time of life.

If I am fat or thin, will my body type influence when I experience menopause?

Yes. If you are extremely thin, you will have a greater chance of going through an earlier menopause compared to someone who is overweight. The body's fatty tissue is capable of converting male hormones (called androgens), produced after menopause by the ovaries and adrenal glands, into estrogen. Generally speaking, if you have more body fat you will produce more estrogen and experience fewer menopausal symptoms. Consequently, women who are more obese will go through menopause later in life. (This statement should not be used as an excuse to gain weight, however, as the consequences of obesity are worse than the symptoms of estrogen deprivation! It is easier to take estrogen replacement after menopause than to lose weight.)

Will the amount of estrogen produced by my body fat and adrenal glands be enough to prevent me from having menopausal symptoms?

It will not allow you to continue menstruating, but it may be sufficient to prevent you from developing hot flashes, vaginal dryness, bladder symptoms, osteoporosis and other menopausal symtoms.

Does the age at which I had my first menstrual period (menarche) influence when I will undergo menopause?

It was first thought that if you had an early menarche, menopause would arrive early, as well. Recent studies have shown, however, no correlation between the ages of menarche and menopause.

If my mother had an early menopause, will that happen to me, too?

Genetics certainly have an influence. There appears to be a tendency for early or late menopause to run in families. If your mother and sisters went through an early menopause, you may do the same.

Has the age at which menopause occurs changed over the years?

Writings dating back to the time of Aristotle and Hippocrates (300-400 B.C.), show menopause occurring in the same general age range (between 40-50) as it does today. Chances are that your grandmothers and their relatives experienced menopause at about the same age as you. But life expectancy was much shorter years ago than it is today. Now, you can anticipate living at least one-third of your life after your menopause.

Will the fact that I took oral contraceptives (birth control pills), influence when I experience menopause?

Studies are just beginning to explore the relationship between birth control pills and menopause. Preliminary evidence does not indicate that the use of birth control pills delays the onset of menopause. The pill, however, if taken well into the later 40's can disguise menopause, since the hormones in the pill will artificially bring on uterine bleeding and prevent menopausal symptoms.

Will my tubal ligation influence when I experience menopause?

In a small number of cases, some types of tubal sterilization procedures may interfere with the blood supply to the ovaries. As a result, the compromised blood supply may cause a premature aging of the ovaries resulting in an earlier menopause.

SURGICAL MENOPAUSE

If I had a hysterectomy, will it influence if and when I have menopausal symptoms?

A hysterectomy is the surgical removal of the uterus and not the ovaries; therefore, it should not result in menopausal symptoms other than the immediate cessation of your menstrual periods. Occasionally, when a hysterectomy is performed, however, the blood supply to the ovaries may be temporarily compromised, interrupting estrogen production by the ovaries and causing hot flashes immediately after surgery. Several years later, the onset of other menopausal symptoms may occur at a slightly earlier age because of this compromised blood supply.

What is surgical menopause?

Surgical menopause occurs when the ovaries are removed surgically for medical reasons such as ovarian tumors, severe pelvic infections, or endometriosis before the natural onset of menopause. The operation is called a *bilateral oophorectomy*. If you are between the ages of 40 and 50 and in need of a hysterectomy, your doctor may discuss the possibility of removing your ovaries along with the uterus (even if the ovaries are normal) to prevent future problems with ovarian cysts and ovarian cancer.

How soon after the removal of my ovaries will I develop menopausal symptoms?

Vasomotor symptoms such as hot flashes, palpitations, and night sweats may occur within a few days of the bilateral oophorectomy. Vaginal dryness usually takes several years to develop but some women who undergo a surgical menopause experience this discomfort within a few months. These menopausal symptoms can be prevented by starting estrogen replacement therapy immediately after surgery.

Is surgical menopause more difficult to go through than a natural menopause?

It can be. The symptoms that result from surgical menopause may begin more abruptly than those of natural menopause because the hormonal disruption is sudden rather than gradual. Estrogen replacement therapy is usually started immediately after a bilateral oophorectomy to prevent hot flashes and other menopausal symptoms. There is some recent evidence, however, that women who undergo surgical menopause do experience some lingering disability, even as much as nine to twelve months after surgery, as compared with women whose menopause occurs naturally. This may be due partially to the sudden decrease in testosterone production by the ovaries, as well as the decrease in estrogen production.

How can I tell if I have reached menopause?

Usually, symptoms such as hot flashes, night sweats, sleep disturbances, and lack of energy will be present. Your physician may check your hormone blood levels of FSH or estradiol. However, many women's hormones fluctuate tremendously during this transition, going from normal levels to levels indicating menopause and then back to normal again. This condition is not uncommon; it is as if you were going in and out of menopause.

Is it better if I have an earlier or later menopause?

Although you may hope to go through an early menopause because you are tired of having menstrual periods, there are advantages to having a later menopause. Symptoms such as skin wrinkling, vaginal and bladder atrophy, osteoporosis, and the possibility of cardiovascular disease will be delayed if you experience a later menopause.

Are there any disadvantages to having a late menopause?

Many women consider the nuisance of having ongoing menstrual periods a disadvantage. A potentially serious consequence of late menopause is a slightly higher incidence of ovarian, breast, and uterine lining (endometrial) cancer. Some types of female cancer are thought to be influenced by estrogen. Their occurrence may be partially related to how many years you have been menstruating.

MALE "MENOPAUSE"

Do men go through menopause?

Possibly. Men do not experience a sudden decrease in production of sex hormones, but they may experience a mid-life crisis which usually has a psychological rather than a hormonal basis. Some researchers have referred to this mid-life crisis as the male "menopause," but it usually occurs around the age of 40 rather than 50. Men do go through an aging process, however, in which they may encounter difficulty performing sexually, but they don't totally lose their ability to produce children until very late in life. The research on male "menopause" and its significance is approximately 20 years behind the study of the female menopause. On the other hand, some researchers have identified a type of male "menopause" they call andropause.

What is andropause?

Andropause refers to the gradual decrease in the male hormones (androgens) as a man ages. Testosterone is the major androgen and during this time, men experience a decrease in blood testosterone levels as well as an associated increase in luteinizing hormone (because of the negative feedback mechanism in the pituitary gland). (See Chapter 2.) Andropause typically manifests itself in men, usually over 60. The symptoms include difficulty maintaining erections, hot flashes, an increase in tiredness, and sleep disturbances. As we have seen, many of these same symptoms are also associated with the female menopause. Yet despite these changes, some men are capable of fathering children when they are well into their 70s and 80s. Testosterone treatment may be tried in some men.

2

What Causes Menopause?

To fully understand menopause, you'll need to grasp the workings of the female reproductive system. This, however, is not easy. Your menstrual period is the end result of a sequence of events that involve the reproductive organs (the uterus and ovaries) as well as the hypothalamus and pituitary glands located in the brain. Most people don't associate these endocrine glands with reproduction, but they are as important as your uterus and ovaries to that process. This chapter explains how the entire system works.

THE ENDOCRINE GLANDS

What is an endocrine gland?

An endocrine gland is an organ that secretes hormones into the bloodstream to influence metabolism and other body processes. The endocrine glands related to the female reproductive system are the ovaries, the pituitary and the hypothalamus glands. The thyroid and adrenal glands also play a role in the functioning of the female reproductive system.

What is a hormone?

A hormone is a chemical substance produced by an endo-crine gland. It is like a "messenger" that tells the cells in your body's organs what to do. The hormone passes directly into the bloodstream and is carried to other organs or tissues where it modifies their structure or function.

What is the hypothalamus?

The hypothalamus is a region in the center of the brain that controls many bodily functions. It slowly matures during childhood, causing the reproductive system to develop. This gland secretes a hormone called *gonadotropin releasing hormone* (GnRH) which stimulates the pituitary gland to secrete its hormones, *follicle stimulating hormone* (FSH) and *luteinizing hormone* (LH). These, in turn, stimulate the ovaries to produce *estrogen* and *progesterone*. All of these hormones, so essential to female reproduction, will be explained.

Does the hypothalamus have other functions?

Yes, it does. The hypothalamus also regulates body temperature. In fact, researchers feel it is the area in the brain that is responsible for causing hot flashes and night sweats when the production of estrogen decreases at the time of menopause. One theory holds that the repeated, pulsating release of GnRH, FSH, and LH from the hypothalamus and pituitary glands actually brings on the hot flash.

What is the role of the pituitary gland?

The pituitary is a pea-sized gland located at the base of the brain, between and behind the eyes. An area in the pituitary gland receives messages from the hypothalamus through GnRH, and then sends *follicle stimulating hormone* (FSH) and

Figure 2-1

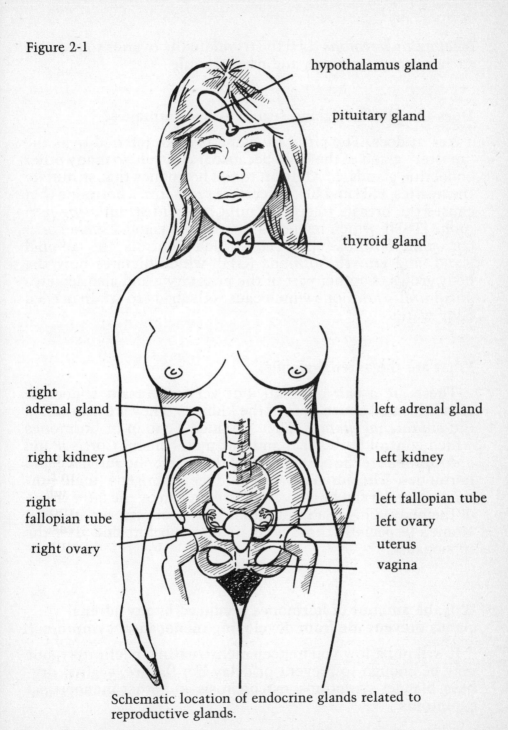

hypothalamus gland

pituitary gland

thyroid gland

right adrenal gland

left adrenal gland

right kidney

left kidney

right fallopian tube

left fallopian tube

left ovary

right ovary

uterus

vagina

Schematic location of endocrine glands related to reproductive glands.

luteinizing hormone (LH) to stimulate the ovaries to produce its hormones, estrogen and progesterone.

Does the pituitary gland secrete other hormones?

Yes, it does. The pituitary gland is often referred to as the "master" gland of the body because it controls so many other endocrine glands. In addition to the hormones that stimulate the ovaries, FSH and LH, it secretes *prolactin,* a hormone that causes the breasts to secrete milk; *thyroid stimulating hormone* (TSH), which regulates the thyroid gland; *adrenocorticotrophic hormone* (ACTH), which controls the adrenal gland; and *growth hormone* (GH), which dictates how the body grows. Another part of the pituitary gland also secretes *antidiuretic hormone* which causes the body to retain needed body water.

What are the adrenal glands?

These are a pair of small, but very important endocrine glands located above each of the kidneys. They are also called the *suprarenal glands.* They produce a group of hormones which control both sugar and salt metabolism. *Cortisol* and *aldosterone* are the best known of the metabolic adrenal gland hormones. The adrenals also produce androgens (male hormones) which can be converted to estrogen by the fatty tissue of the body. This is an important source of estrogen in some women (especially those who are obese) before and after the menopause.

Will the amount of hormones produced by my adrenal glands prevent me from developing menopausal symptoms?

It will not allow you to keep menstruating indefinitely, but may be enough to prevent or delay hot flashes, vaginal dryness, bladder symptoms, osteoporosis and other menopausal symptoms.

THE REPRODUCTIVE ORGANS AND HORMONES

What is the uterus?

The uterus is an upside down, pear-shaped, three layered muscular organ that serves as an incubator and home for a developing pregnancy. It consists of a flattened body called the *corpus* with a cylindrical shaped neck called the *cervix*. The cervix is often referred to as the "mouth" of the uterus. It opens during labor to allow the baby to be delivered. The cervix protrudes into the vagina. Its surface is the area scraped during a pap smear.

What tissues make up the uterus?

The body of the uterus consists of three layers:

- **a thin, smooth outer surface called the *serosa***
- **a middle thick, muscular layer called the *myometrium***
- **and an inner lining called the *endometrium***

The myometrium or muscular layer makes up most of the body of the uterus.

What is the purpose of the endometrium?

The endometrium, or uterine lining, receives a fertilized egg and provides nourishment for the developing embryo during the first few weeks of pregnancy. It is the part of the uterus that is shed during a menstrual period.

What are the ovaries?

Women have two ovaries, one on each side of the uterus. These are the sex glands, having three functions; the development of eggs (ova); the production of the female hormones,

Chart 2-1

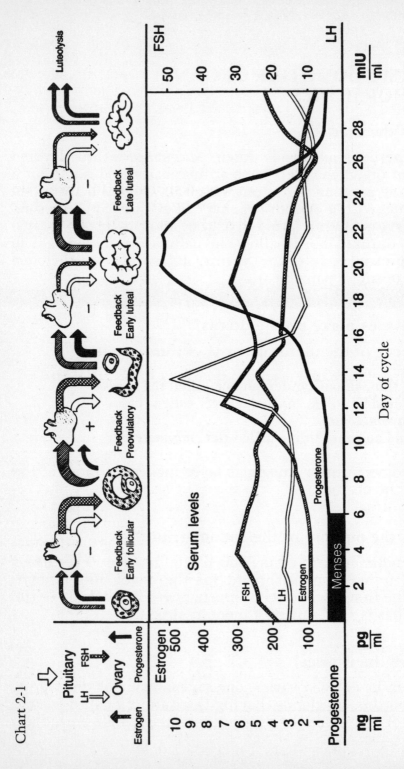

Relationship of the pituitary hormones FSH and LH to the production of estrogen and progesterone during a normal menstrual cycle.

estrogen and progesterone; and the development of lesser amounts of the male hormone, testosterone. The ovaries are stimulated to do their tasks by the pituitary hormones, FSH and LH.

What is estrogen?

Estrogen is the female hormone responsible for breast development and menstruation. Your ovaries actually produce several kinds of estrogen: estrone, estradiol, and estriol.

Are there sources of estrogen other than my ovaries?

Yes, the adrenal glands secrete small amounts of estrogen and other hormones (androgens) that are converted to estrogen by the body fat. The ovaries also produce small amounts of androgens which can be converted to estrogen by the body fat.

How do the pituitary and ovarian hormones interact with each other?

FSH and estrogen work by a circular process called the *negative-feedback loop*: when FSH is secreted by the pituitary gland, it causes an increase in production of estrogen from the ovaries. The rise in estrogen, however, causes a *decrease* in production of FSH. This decrease, in turn, results in a decreased estrogen production. That triggers an *increase* in FSH, and the cycle repeats itself from the top. The chart on page 18 shows the fine balance established between these hormones during a normal menstrual cycle. A physician often uses a blood test to check your level of FSH, to determine if you are in menopause. An FSH reading of more than 40 (milli–international units per milliliter) indicates menopause.

What is progesterone?

Progesterone is the ovarian hormone that prepares the uterine lining for implantation of a fertilized egg. If you do not become pregnant during the menstrual cycle, the progesterone level in your blood falls off quickly and causes the uterine lining to shed. That shedding is called the menstrual period.

OVULATION

What is the ovum?

The *ovum* is the female reproductive cell also called the egg. It grows and develops within the *Graafian follicle* in the ovary. The ovum is expelled from the ovary at the time of ovulation. When fertilized by the sperm, it develops into an embryo, then a fetus and finally a baby.

What is ovulation?

Ovulation is the process by which the egg separates from the follicle and is expelled from the ovary and picked up by the Fallopian tube. If conception occurs, it usually takes place within the Fallopian tube with subsequent implantation in the uterine cavity.

What are Graafian follicles?

Graaffian follicles are small cystic structures within the ovary in which the eggs develop. The follicles have two main functions: to ripen and prepare an egg for ovulation and to produce estrogen. Special cells within the follicle are the main source of estrogen produced by the body.

What roles do FSH and LH play in ovulation?

The pituitary hormone FSH travels through the bloodstream and stimulates the Graafian follicle to develop and prepare an egg for ovulation. Approximately 12-36 hours prior to ovulation, a slight surge in estrogen occurs stimulating a sudden increase in the production of *luteinizing hormone* (LH) from the pituitary gland. This causes the egg to be expelled from the ovary.

How many follicles do the ovaries contain?

Interestingly, at five months of gestation, there are approximately 700,000 follicles in a female fetus. At birth, the ovaries contain approximately 400,000 follicles. By the age of 40, the ovaries only contain about 5,000 to 10,000 follicles with the number rapidly decreasing after that. At menopause, only a few follicles remain. They become unresponsive to the hormones (FSH and LH) produced by the pituitary gland.

If I only ovulate one egg a month, what happens to the other follicles during my lifetime?

You will ovulate approximately 400-450 eggs during your menstruating years (about one a month for 35 to 40 years). Although each follicle contains an egg, most fail to fully develop. The underdeveloped follicles and eggs simply disintegrate within the ovary (*atresia*). Developing follicles produce estrogen, but once they dissolve, they no longer do so.

What if more than one follicle matures in a month?

If two follicles mature and each expels an egg which becomes fertilized, fraternal (non-identical) twins will result. In fact, the main purpose of the ovarian stimulating agents used to resolve infertility such as Clomid, Serophene, Pergonal and Metrodin, is to stimulate the Graafian follicle within the ovary to produce eggs. If the ovaries are overstimulated, you may ovulate several eggs, resulting in multiple births!

Do both ovaries function each month?

Although both ovaries contain developing Graafian follicles, usually only one follicle within one ovary becomes dominant during each menstrual cycle. The ovaries do not alternate ovulation on a regular basis: you may ovulate from your right ovary for several months in a row; then the left one takes over.

If I have only one ovary, will I ovulate every other month?

No, even if you have one ovary, ovulation will occur every month, and you will have monthly menstrual cycles. The remaining ovary receives the stimulation from the pituitary hormones, FSH and LH, and develops a mature follicle each month.

What is the corpus luteum?

The *corpus luteum* is a yellow mass of cells formed within the Graafian follicle after it expels the egg. Actually, after ovulation the Graafian follicle *becomes* a corpus luteum.

Figure 2-2

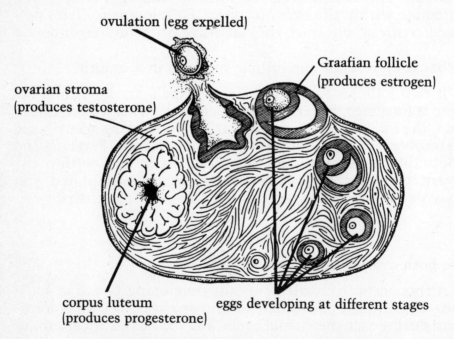

Ovulation occurring in the ovary with developing eggs and a corpus luteum.

What is the purpose of the corpus luteum?

The corpus luteum secretes the hormone progesterone which prepares the uterine lining for pregnancy. If you were to become pregnant, the corpus luteum would persist and continue to produce progesterone to support the uterine lining for the growing pregnancy. At about 12 weeks of gestation, the placenta produces enough progesterone to support the pregnancy and the corpus luteum slowly dissolves. Occasionally, the corpus luteum of pregnancy becomes enlarged, causing a corpus luteal ovarian cyst which may cause pain during the first few months of pregnancy.

If pregnancy does not occur, the corpus luteum lasts only 14 days, then gradually dissolves and becomes a *corpus albicans* (a dried up, non-functioning scar within the ovary).

What if I do not become pregnant during a menstrual cycle?

Your uterine lining will shed as the progesterone level decreases. The shedding of the uterine lining each month is called menstruation.

MENSTRUATION

What causes the build-up and shedding of the endometrium each month?

Estrogen causes the build-up of the uterine lining. When you ovulate, the corpus luteum produces progesterone which gives the uterine lining a "lush" appearance and prepares it for implantation. If pregnancy does not occur, the progesterone level in your blood falls off quite rapidly as the corpus luteum has a limited life span (14 days), resulting in menstruation. The uterine lining sheds because progesterone is responsible for "supporting" it. When progesterone production suddenly falls, the uterine lining cannot sustain itself.

What controls the menstrual cycle?

The hormones of the hypothalamus (GnRH) control those of the pituitary (FSH and LH) which, in turn, regulate the ovarian hormones, estrogen and progesterone. All of these glands and hormones (called the *hypothalamic-pituitary-ovarian axis*) must be synchronized for you to experience normal menstrual periods. Anything that interferes with the hypothalamus (such as stress), the pituitary gland (small tumors called *microadenomas*), or the ovaries (ovarian failure and menopause) may cause a delay in or an abnormal menstrual period.

THE MATURATION AND THE AGING OF THE REPRODUCTIVE SYSTEM

When does the process begin that leads to menopause?

The process leading to menopause actually begins with the development of the reproductive organs during puberty. The organs become functionally operative and secondary sex characteristics develop during your late childhood and early teenage years.

At what age does puberty start?

The average age for the onset of menstruation is 12-1/2, with 90% of girls menstruating by the age of 15.

What happened to my body when I went through puberty?

The sequence of events is usually predictable. One of the first signs of impending puberty is a reaccumulation of the "baby fat" that was present in the first few years of life and then disappeared between the ages of four and eight. The age at which this change occurs varies greatly with each person. A girl may start to reaccumulate her "baby fat" as early as age eight or nine. This fat is deposited in the *subcutaneous* tissues, giving a girl a filled out, rather plump appearance. About a year after the fat deposits occur, a growth spurt is initiated. The pelvic bones widen and hips develop. This is usually followed by the development of breasts, then pubic and underarm (*axillary*) hair. The growth spurt now accelerates, leading to the final event: menstruation. It usually takes two years from the first sign of breast development to the onset of menstruation.

What causes puberty?

The hypothalamus starts to mature and secretes *gonadotropin-releasing hormone* (GnRH). This travels by way of the bloodstream and stimulates certain cells within the pituitary gland to secrete two of its main hormones: *follicle stimulating hormone* (FSH) and *luteinizing hormone* (LH). FSH stimulates the follicles within the ovaries to produce estrogen, followed by a surge in LH which triggers ovulation and the production of progesterone. Estrogen is the main female hormone responsible for the events around puberty— fat reaccumulation, the growth spurt, breast development and menstruation.

Is there a hormonal similarity between puberty and menopause?

Surprisingly, there is. As a young girl, it may have taken several years for your periods to become regular. This was due to the immaturity of the hypothalamic-pituitary-ovarian axis: the glands were not fully synchronized with each other. If you had irregular periods during your adolescence, you were probably not ovulating regularly and may have had several periods that were very heavy and seemed like they would never end.

The same mechanism affects the hypothalamic-pituitary-ovarian axis in perimenopausal women, as well. Periods become irregular and heavy and may be spaced further apart with an occasionally missed cycle. This is due to the aging of ovaries and the interruption of the normal relationship between the glands. You do not ovulate regularly, and the consequent irregular periods are due to sporadic estrogen and progesterone secretion, due in turn to aging of the hypothalamic-pituitary-ovarian axis.

What happens to FSH, estrogen, and progesterone at menopause?

During the menstrual years, the production of FSH from the pituitary gland and estrogen from the ovaries are in balance. When you approach menopause, however, the follicles within the ovaries are no longer capable of producing sufficient estrogen, despite the increased level of FSH production. Since there is no estrogen to feed back on the pituitary, the FSH level remains at a persistently high level. *This persistent elevation of FSH is one of the tests your doctor may perform to determine if your ovaries have stopped producing estrogen and you are in menopause.*

Progesterone is the hormone produced by the corpus luteum of the ovary after ovulation occurs. *You must ovulate to produce progesterone.* This is a very important fact to remember when we discuss the abnormal bleeding that can occur during the menopausal period.

ANOVULATION AND MENOPAUSE

What does the term "ovarian failure" mean?

"Ovarian failure is another term for menopause. It is the failure of the ovaries to produce estrogen.

What happens to my menstrual cycles during the years before menopause?

When some women enter their 40's, estrogen production from the follicles may become sporadic, disturbing the balance that had been established between all of the reproductive hormones. As a result of this imbalance, ovulation ceases,

Chart 2-2

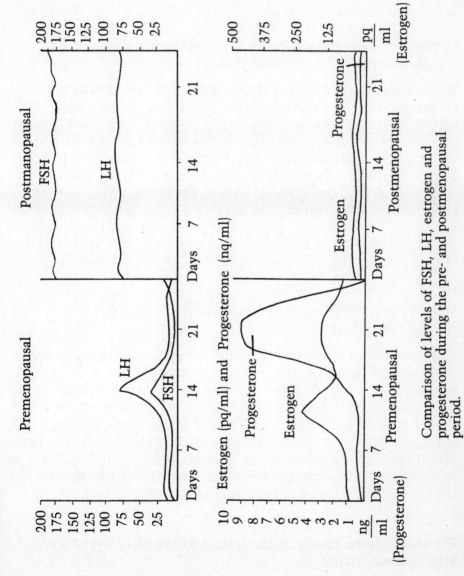

Comparison of levels of FSH, LH, estrogen and progesterone during the pre- and postmenopausal period.

even though the ovaries continue to produce estrogen. This causes irregular menstrual periods.

Is there a danger in having a constant estrogen stimulation to the uterine lining?

Yes. If you are producing estrogen but not ovulating, your uterus is under a constant stimulus from the estrogen without benefit of progesterone. If this persists long enough (usually longer than six months), it could lead to one of several different conditions called *endometrial hyperplasia, atypical endometrial hyperplasia,* or even cancer of the uterine lining (*endometrial cancer*). All of these disorders are potentially serious. Sampling the uterine lining with biopsies, aspirations, or a D & C is necessary to explain unusual menstrual bleeding in the perimenopausal period. I will discuss these issues in more detail in Chapters 3 and 12.

How is anovulation (not ovulating) similar to taking estrogen?

If you are not ovulating, you are not producing progesterone. This would be the same as taking estrogen on a daily basis without the progesterone. Your uterine lining will be under continual stimulation of estrogen either from your own ovaries or from the estrogen pills. Endometrial hyperplasia, a typical hyperplasia or uterine lining cancer may all develop from either of these circumstances. This is why progesterone is usually given to women who still have their uterus and are taking estrogen replacement during the menopause.

Do all women produce the same amount of estrogen after menopause?

No, they do not. Estrogen production varies from woman to woman. It depends on a number of factors, including body fat. Some women continue to produce significant amounts of estrogen after menopause, while other women produce very little.

3

What's Happening To My Menstrual Cycles?

Many subtle changes occur during the climacteric—the ten years preceding menopause. If you are in your late 30's or early 40's, you may have noticed a change in your menstrual cycle. Your periods may now be irregular and/or associated with episodes of very heavy bleeding. These may be the first signs that you are approaching the premenopausal phase even though you are not having the typical hot flashes associated with menopause.

CHANGES IN MENSTRUAL PATTERNS

What might be the first sign that I am entering the climacteric?

Usually you'll note a change in the intervals between or the length of your periods. You may also suddenly find cramps a problem. Occasionally, hot flashes may occur even though you are having regular menstrual periods.

What happens to the pattern of my menstrual cycles over the years?

The bleeding pattern following your first menstrual cycle (at menarche) is often irregular. Some of the cycles during your adolescence may be unusually short or long. Between the ages of 20-40, menstrual cycles are usually regular, with a clocklike predictable pattern of both interval and length. Around the age of 40, however, the cycles again may return to a pattern of irregularity, similar to the years following the menarche.

What is considered a normal menstrual cycle?

The interval between menstrual cycles is calculated from the first day of menstrual flow to the first day of the next menstrual flow. This interval is 26-34 days in most women, with the majority in the 28-32 day range. The total length of your menstrual flow will vary from three to seven days, including any pre- or post-menstrual spotting.

I've had irregular periods all of my life. Is this unusual?

No, it is not. Some women never get into a pattern of regular 28-32 day cycles. They have very sporadic and irregular periods every two to four months without a predictable pattern. This *oligomenorrhea* is caused by an unsynchronized hypothalamic-pituitary-ovarian axis (See Chapter 2). If you decide to become pregnant, you may need help with one of the stimulating drugs to induce ovulation because you are only ovulating a few times a year. Most women with oligomenorrhea continue in the same menstrual pattern most of their lives, or they may experience regular cycles for a few years and then return to a pattern of irregularity.

If I have irregular cycles, will I begin menopause at a different time?

No. You will undergo menopause at the same age as other women.

How common is it for a disturbance in hormones to cause irregular periods?

If you are past the age of 40, studies have shown that as many as 30%-50% of your cycles may be associated with abnormal production of estrogen and progesterone. This also explains why fertility is decreased in women over 35— hormone production from the ovaries becomes less predictable.

Will my periods become irregular prior to menopause?

That depends. You may notice a change in your menstrual cycles prior to menopause, but not so much that you need medical attention. I would like to emphasize that *most* women go through the menopausal years with little difficulty with their periods.

If you do experience some irregularity, typically you may only notice your periods being further apart. At first the normal cycle interval may extend to five or six week intervals, then to every other or once every third month. Eventually the periods stop. Alternatively, your periods may become irregular and unpredictable. The interval between cycles may shorten to 21-24 days with occasional cycles occuring at two week intervals. Or, you may continue to have regular cycles until your last period. Looking back on it 12 months later, you may realize that you have already gone through menopause. Other symptoms, such as hot flashes and vaginal dryness, may or may not be present along with the irregular menses.

Will the amount of menstrual flow also change?

Most women will notice a lighter flow as they approach menopause. It is possible, however, for the flow to become extremely heavy and marked by passage of large clots even though you never had them previously. Prolonged pre- and post-menstrual staining and spotting may also occur. Indeed, you may feel you are bleeding more during the month than not. The entire cycle of spotting-flow-spotting may go on for 10 to 14 days or more. Occasionally, one period appears to run into another. The heavy flow with the passage of clots can be so distressing that you fear leaving home or going on a trip during the first few days of your period. Some of the clots may be as large as your fist.

HEAVY BLEEDING

How do I know if I should be concerned about the amount of flow I am having?

What you consider heavy menstrual bleeding may be fairly normal for someone else. The change in the pattern you have been used to is what is important. You should be aware that your periods have suddenly changed and should discuss it with your physician.

What are signs of heavy bleeding?

The total flow is considered heavy if you soak through a full-thickness sanitary pad from one side to the other and have to change that pad more than once per hour. Soaking through tampons plus full thickness pads can also be considered heavy if you have to change them at least once per hour. Occasionally, the flow becomes so heavy you will soak through tampons and pads. If the type and amount of bleeding concern you, consult your physician.

Do other symptoms accompany excessive flow?

Symptoms which may indicate that you are bleeding heavily include light-headedness, weakness, chills, sweating, or a cold, clammy feeling.

HORMONAL IMBALANCES AND DYSFUNCTIONAL UTERINE BLEEDING

What causes the changes in my menstrual cycle?

A hormonal disturbance or a uterine abnormality can cause changes in your menstrual cycle during the climacteric.

What is abnormal menstrual bleeding called?

The most common cause for abnormal bleeding in the perimenopausal period is *dysfunctional uterine bleeding.* This abnormality is caused by the ovaries' irregular production of estrogen and progesterone. It does not stem from a problem within the uterus.

What causes the hormonal changes during the perimenopausal years?

As discussed in the previous chapter, the hypothalamus and pituitary glands in the brain control your ovaries. As you approach your 40's, your ovaries begin to run out of eggs: the production of estrogen becomes sporadic and ovulation is triggered only irregularly. The decrease in estrogen production interferes with the balance of the negative feedback mechanism between estrogen, FSH and LH. The decrease in estrogen production along with its failure to trigger LH release and ovulation is the main cause for the change in your menstrual cycle. If you stop ovulating, your ovaries stop producing progesterone.

What happens to my uterine lining if I don't ovulate?

Two things may occur: you may either bleed too much or you may go several months without a period. If you don't ovulate, you will not produce progesterone or shed your uterine lining on a regular basis. If several months go by without a period, the uterine lining becomes stimulated by a steady secretion of estrogen from the ovaries. Since there is no progesterone to counteract the estrogen build-up, the areas that are under continuous estrogen stimulation outgrow their blood supply and start sloughing and bleeding in a very unpredictable fashion. The uterus becomes confused—parts of it are sloughing while other parts are building up. As a result, the uterus bleeds irregularly, with episodes of prolonged spotting and possibly heavy, gushy periods. The bleeding is very similar to the bleeding that may occur if a woman takes estrogen pills daily for several months in a row without progesterone.

Can stress cause dysfunctional uterine bleeding?

External factors may very easily influence your menstrual periods. The hypothalamic-pituitary-ovarian axis is sensitive to external forces, such as stress, medications, and tranquilizers. In addition, during the perimenopausal years the hormones are more susceptible to changes, so obvious or even subtle stress may indeed have some influence on periods at this time even if it had never caused a problem previously. If you have irregular periods to begin with, you will be even more vulnerable to the external forces which cause irregular cycles or amenorrhea.

Will certain medications cause me to have irregular cycles?

Yes they may. If you are taking any potent tranquilizer such as Mellaril or Thorazine, you may notice your periods becoming irregular or even stopping. Other medications such as cortisone and Acutance may also cause irregular bleeding patterns in some women.

PROGESTERONE THERAPY FOR DYSFUNCTIONAL UTERINE BLEEDING

How can dysfunctional uterine bleeding be treated?

Dysfunctional uterine bleeding can be treated by progesterone therapy.

What is progesterone therapy?

Progesterone therapy simply replaces the progesterone that you normally would have produced if you were ovulating on a regular basis. See your physician if you are having abnormal uterine bleeding. He will perform an examination to determine the cause. If the pelvic examination is normal and there are no gross abnormalities of the uterus, the cause is most likely dysfunctional bleeding.

Your physician may prescribe progesterone pills for 7 to 14 days to counteract the build up of the uterine lining caused by the estrogen. Stopping the progesterone will induce a period. It is the introduction of progesterone to an estrogen-stimulated uterine lining, followed by its abrupt withdrawal, that causes a menstrual flow. If your medical history calls for it, an endometrial biopsy may be advised before you take the progesterone.

How is the progesterone given?

Women usually take progesterone in pills. Several different types of progesterone are available for this purpose: Provera, Amen, Curretabs, or Cycrin. (See Chapter 13 for a discussion of these medications.) The dose is often one or two pills a day for 5 to 15 days depending on the degree and amount of bleeding you are experiencing. For a very heavy flow, the progesterone may be given several times a day for a few days then gradually tapered over additional days. Further bleeding can be expected two to four days following the course of treatment, but this should resemble a more normal menstrual flow. Once you are over this episode of bleeding, your periods should revert to normal unless you fail to ovulate again.

Why will I bleed again after finishing the progesterone?

During a normal menstrual cycle, the ovary's secretion of progesterone lasts only as long as the corpus luteum is present (about 14 days). When the progesterone level drops, bleeding results. The same phenomenon occurs after you take progesterone orally. When you stop after ten days of treatment, the progesterone no longer supports the uterine lining and you bleed.

Does estrogen have to be present in order for progesterone therapy to work ?

Yes, it does. In fact, this is called a *progesterone challenge test* and is used to determine if you have already undergone menopause. After your doctor prescribes progesterone, you know your body is still producing estrogen if you get a period. If, on the other hand, you do not get your period, your ovaries may be producing insufficient estrogen to thicken the uterine lining and you may already be in the menopause.

Are there other reasons why a woman will not get a period after taking progesterone?

Yes, there are. The possibility of pregnancy should be considered during the perimenopausal years when your menstrual cycles become irregular or absent. Absent periods can also result from dysfunction of the hypothalamus gland (called *hypothalamic amenorrhea*). In this case, GnRH is completely suppressed from the hypothalamus. A serum FSH level may be useful to determine if menopause has occurred or if insufficient GnRH is being produced. If the FSH level is low, it means there is no stimulation of the pituitary gland by the hypothalamus to produce FSH. If the FSH level is high, it is a sign of ovarian failure or menopause.

How long should I stay on progesterone therapy for irregular cycles?

This will vary greatly and will depend upon how often and irregularly your bleeding has occurred. In many cases it may be necessary to be on the progesterone for only one cycle. Other times it may be advisable to take a 10-14 day course of progesterone for three to six months at monthly intervals to control your menstrual cycle. After this trial, the progesterone can be stopped to see what your cycles will do on their own. It will be up to your physician to decide what the best treatment is for you.

If I take progesterone, when can I expect my period?

Your period should come within two to four days after taking the last progesterone pill and should resemble a more normal menstrual cycle. If you don't get back on track after the first month, however, don't get discouraged. Often it takes several months for normal menstrual function to return.

How long should I stay on hormonal therapy for abnormally heavy bleeding?

If progesterone therapy is helping control your cycles, there is no harm in continuing with it for several months. After three to six months, you may stop the medication to see what happens without it. Often the hormonal imbalance will have spontaneously resolved itself along with the excessive bleeding. At other times, it may be worthwhile to continue the therapy until you no longer bleed from the progesterone withdrawal. This cessation of menstrual bleeding indicates a lack of estrogen production and the onset of menopause. At this time it may be appropriate to start on combined estrogen and progesterone hormone replacement therapy.

Does progesterone have any side effects?

The side effects of progesterone include abdominal bloating, headaches, breast tenderness, moodiness, and mild fluid retention. If any of these symptoms do occur, the dose can be lowered. Some women are just not able to take progesterone without bothersome side effects. Most however, feel much better when they resume regular menstrual bleeding.

PERSISTENT BLEEDING

What if I continue to bleed irregularly after progesterone therapy?

Any persistent abnormal bleeding must be evaluated by sampling the uterine lining (by endometrial biopsies, an endometrial aspiration, or a D & C) before persisting with progesterone therapy. Progesterone is given to treat hormonal disturbances. It will not help if you have an abnormality within the uterine cavity such as polyps, fibroids or even a malignancy. (See below.) Depending on the degree of abnormal bleeding and how old you are, it may be advisable to perform a biopsy of the uterine lining *before* starting progesterone therapy. Your doctor will know what's best for you.

What if progesterone alone does not help?

Because the exact origin of irregular and heavy menses is not known, different approaches to this problem may be in order before resorting to more radical therapy, such as a hysterectomy. If your periods are just heavy and not irregular, one of the medications that inhibits the hormone *prostaglandin* may be of benefit.

What is prostaglandin?

Prostaglandin is a hormone secreted by the cells of the uterine lining responsible for the severe menstrual cramps that some women experience. Anti-prostaglandin medications such as *ibuprofen* (Motrin, Advil, Nuprin, Medipren) have been shown to cut down on menstrual cramps as well as heavy menstrual bleeding if taken regularly throughout your menstrual cycle. I suggest 400-600mg of ibuprofen three or four times daily at the onset and throughout your period. If the over-the-counter ibuprofen doesn't help, your doctor can prescribe several prostaglandin inhibitors (Anaprox, Ponstel, Meclomen, Naproxen).

Do any other medications help heavy periods?

Some researchers theorize that the uterus' inability to contract and squeeze the small blood vessels causes heavy menstrual bleeding. Medications such as *ergotrate* or *methergine* help constrict the uterine muscle to close off small bleeding vessels. They are usually taken one 0.2mg tablet every four to six hours during the days of heavy menstrual flow. Ergotrate and methergine are often used immediately after childbirth to help the uterus contract and return to normal size.

Do these medications have any side effects?

Since ergotrate and methergine can also constrict the muscle of the blood vessels (vasoconstrictors), you should not take them if you have high blood pressure or evidence of cardiovascular disease. When taken to prevent heavy periods, they may cause cramps more severe than normal. Because of the possible side effects of these medications, they are usually recommended on a short term basis.

OTHER UTERINE ABNORMALITIES THAT CAN CAUSE UNUSUAL BLEEDING

What if none of these measures help the abnormal bleeding?

If progesterone therapy or one of the other medications do not help your heavy or irregular periods, other investigational studies should be performed. A hysteroscopy examination or a D & C may be indicated. If these fail to determine the cause or alleviate the bleeding, a hysterectomy or laser ablation may be indicated. These are discussed in Chapter 12.

If dysfunctional bleeding is not causing the irregular periods what else could be wrong?

Disorders of the uterus itself such as endometrial hyperplasia, fibroids (myomas), polyps, endometriosis, or adenomyosis may cause irregular periods during the perimenopausal period. If pregnancy is a possibility, any complication, such as an ectopic or a threatened or incomplete miscarriage may also cause abnormal bleeding.

ENDOMETRIAL HYPERPLASIA AND ENDOMETRIAL CANCER

What is endometrial hyperplasia?

Endometrial hyperplasia is a condition in which the glands and tissue that make up the uterine lining multiply on themselves to the point that an abnormal number of glands are present. When observed under a microscope, the glands appear to be lying on top of each other rather than separated by the supporting tissue, called the *stroma*.

What causes endometrial hyperplasia?

Unopposed and excessive estrogen stimulation of the uterine lining is the most common cause of endometrial hyperplasia. By "unopposed" estrogen, I mean estrogen without pro-gesterone, as exists with most cases of dysfunctional uterine bleeding. If you do not ovulate and do not produce pro-gesterone, the uterine lining will be under a continuous stimulation of estrogen. This may result in the development of endometrial hyperplasia. Taking estrogen after menopause without progesterone may also lead to endometrial hyperpla-sia, as this is the administration of "unopposed" estrogen. If the continuous stimulation of unopposed estrogen goes on long enough, *atypical endometrial hyperplasia* or even en-dometrial cancer may develop.

What is atypical endometrial hyperplasia?

This condition occurs when the cells within the endometri-al glands take on a "wilder" configuration, resembling a pre-cancerous condition. The central part of the cell (called the nucleus) becomes larger and the endometrial glands, them-selves, become more twisted and irregular. Endometrial hyperplasia is a benign condition, but many physicians con-sider atypical endometrial hyperplasia to be precancerous.

What is endometrial cancer?

Endometrial cancer is a further extension of atypical en-dometrial hyperplasia. The endometrial glands actually start invading the supporting tissue around the uterus (the en-dometrial *stroma*). If the glands spread outside the uterus, metastatic cancer is present. This can interfere with the func-tion of the vital organs, such as the brain, liver, or lungs, resulting in death.

What are the symptoms of endometrial hyperplasia, atypical endometrial hyperplasia, and endometrial cancer?

Abnormal uterine bleeding is the most common symptom of these conditions. That is why it is important to explain any abnormal menstrual bleeding during the perimenopausal and postmenopausal years with a sampling of the uterine lining. (I discuss this later in this chapter and in Chapter 12.)

Are certain women more prone to endometrial hyperplasia and endometrial cancer?

Yes, women who do not ovulate regularly and who have only a few periods a year are more prone to hyperplasia because they are not producing progesterone to counteract the uterine lining build-up caused by estrogen. Women who are very obese are also more prone to these conditions. Their body fat converts androgens to estrogen as if they were taking continuous estrogen by mouth. Women taking estrogen replacement therapy without progesterone will also have a higher incidence of these diseases.

What is the treatment for endometrial hyperplasia?

The uterine lining should be sampled using a biopsy, aspiration, or D & C to explain any perimenopausal or postmenopausal abnormal bleeding. If endometrial hyperplasia exists, the treatment is the replacement of the missing hormone— progesterone. If you are not ovulating regularly, a 10- to 14-day course of progesterone should be prescribed periodically (about every 8 to 12 weeks) to induce a menstrual period and the sloughing of the uterine lining. A D & C will often cause the uterine lining to temporarily revert to normal. If abnormal bleeding persists after medical treatment, endometrial ablation or a hysterectomy may be necessary. (See Chapter 12.)

How is atypical endometrial hyperplasia treated?

Since atypical endometrial hyperplasia is a precancerous condition, a hysterectomy is often recommended if you no longer wish to have children. Progesterone therapy may be tried for several months under very close observation and follow-up if you don't want or are not a candidate for a hysterectomy. Resampling the uterine lining with a D & C after a few months of progesterone to make sure the atypical hyperplasia has not progressed to actual cancer is a must if progesterone therapy is used.

How is endometrial cancer treated?

The treatment for endometrial cancer depends on the stage of the cancer. Most endometrial cancers are found early. In that case, a hysterectomy with the removal of both ovaries and tubes will give excellent results. Radiation therapy or chemotherapy may have to be added if the cancer is not found at the earliest stage. Biopsy of the pelvic and abdominal lymph nodes may be necessary at the time of surgery to determine if the cancer has spread.

FIBROID TUMORS (MYOMA)

What are uterine fibroids?

Fibroids are the second most common cause of irregular bleeding during the perimenopausal years. Fibroid tumors of the uterus are a benign growth of the uterine muscle. The medical terms for fibroids are *leiomyomas* or *myomas*.

Figure 3-1

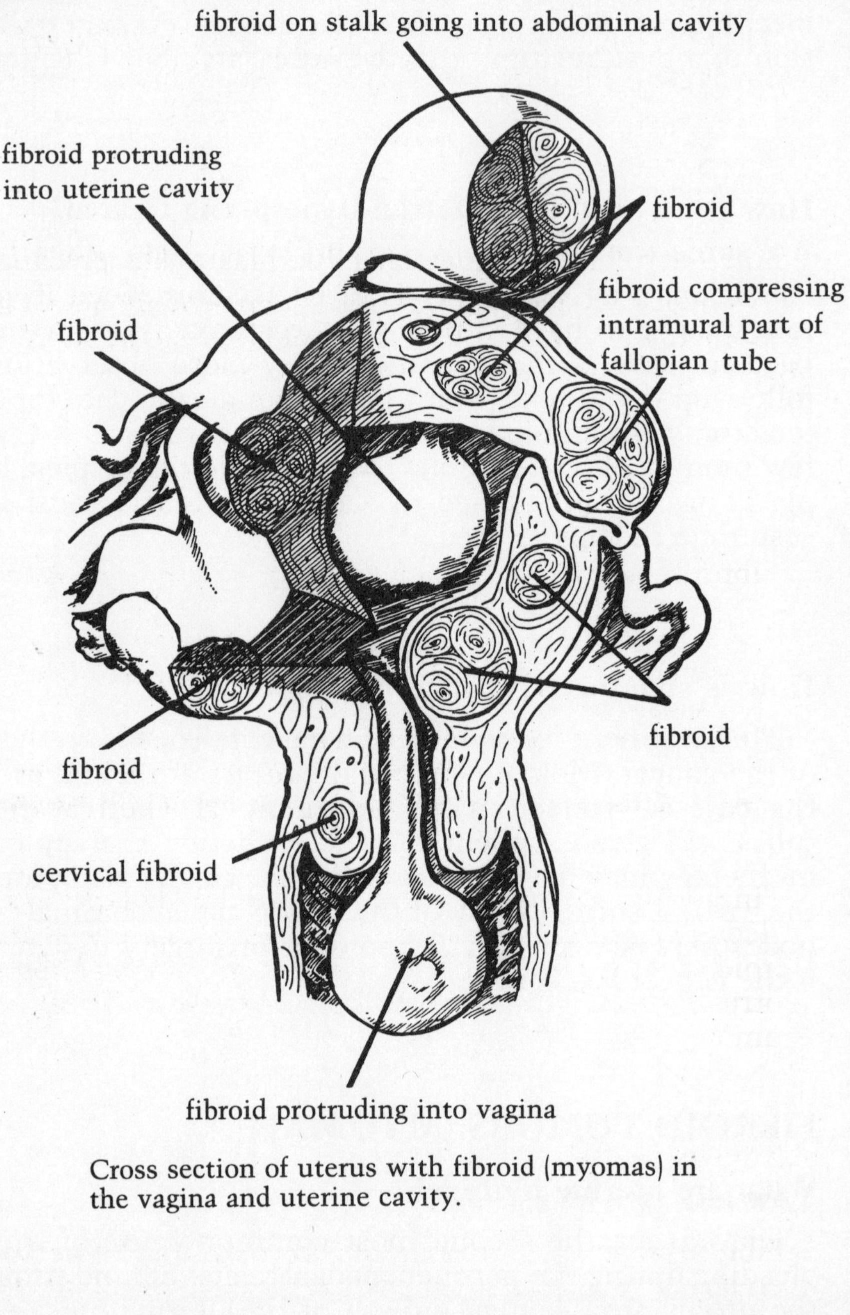

fibroid on stalk going into abdominal cavity

fibroid protruding into uterine cavity

fibroid

fibroid

fibroid

fibroid compressing intramural part of fallopian tube

fibroid

cervical fibroid

fibroid protruding into vagina

Cross section of uterus with fibroid (myomas) in the vagina and uterine cavity.

How common are fibroids?

They are very common, with as many as 20%-30% of *all* women over the age of 30 having some evidence of fibroids.

Are some woman more prone to fibroids than others?

Yes. Black women have a much higher incidence of fibroid tumors than white women. Fibroids occur in as many as 50%-60% of black women.

Where do fibroids grow in the uterus?

Fibroids may grow in three different locations in the uterus.

- *Subserosal* or *subperitoneal* fibroids occur on the external surface of the uterus protruding into the abdominal cavity.
- *Intramural fibroids* grow within the wall of the uterus totally surrounded by normal uterine tissue.
- *Submucosal* or *submucous* fibroids protrude into the uterine cavity.

Finally, some fibroids grow at the end of a stalk. These are called *pedunculated subserosal* or *pedunculated submucosal* fibroids. Occasionally, a pedunculated submucosal fibroid can protrude through the cervical canal and is seen during a pelvic exam.

How large are fibroids?

Fibroids may vary from the size of a pea to a basketball and even larger! Most of the time when they can be felt on a pelvic exam, they are about the size of a golf ball.

What causes fibroids?

Nobody knows for sure, but they are under the influence of the ovarian hormone, estrogen. Estrogen or an estrogen/ progesterone imbalance which occurs during the perimeno- pausal years may cause fibroids that have remained stable and have been present for a number of years to suddenly start growing. During the premenopausal years fibroids can sud- denly start to cause symptoms. Once you have reached meno- pause and have stopped producing estrogen, the fibroid should shrink. A benign fibroid tumor should never form or grow before a girl starts her periods or after the menopause.

What are the symptoms of fibroids?

The symptoms will depend on the tumor's size and loca- tion. Most women who have fibroids *will not* experience any symptoms. If you do have symptoms, abnormal bleeding is the most common. Fibroids within the muscle of the uterus (in- tramural) may prevent the uterus from constricting at the time of a period causing extremely heavy bleeding. Heavy menstrual bleeding may also occur if fibroids are located on the surface of the uterine lining (submucous), even if they are quite small (the size of a pea). If fibroids become large enough, they may cause pressure or heaviness in the pelvis and lower abdomen, pressure on the rectum resulting in constipation, or pressure on the bladder, causing urinary frequency.

Can fibroids cause pain?

Most fibroids do not cause pain. However, if a fibroid is on a stalk (as in a pedunculated subserous fibroid) and protrudes into the abdominal cavity, it may twist and cut off its own blood supply causing sudden, sharp abdominal pain. A rapidly enlarging fibroid may also cause pain if it outgrows its own blood supply and degenerates. This condition is called red degeneration or *necrosis* of a fibroid tumor. The pain from either the twisting (*torsion*) or degeneration may be severe enough to require emergency surgery.

Are fibroids dangerous?

The vast majority of fibroids are benign and not dangerous if they do not cause symptoms. Rarely, especially if a fibroid grows extemely rapidly, it may be a sign that it is developing into a uterine cancer called a *uterine sarcoma.* The malignant degeneration of a fibroid is uncommon, but if your fibroid suddenly starts growing rapidly, it should be removed to make sure it hasn't undergone such a dangerous change.

How are fibroids diagnosed?

Your physician diagnoses most fibroids during your yearly pelvic examination and pap smear. He can usually tell if fibroids are present when he does the bimanual part of the pelvic exam (where he places one hand in the vagina and places the other hand on your abdomen to feel for abnormalities of the uterus or ovaries). The uterus may feel irregular and bumpy. It is important to differentiate a fibroid from another pelvic mass such as an ovarian cyst or tumor. Submucous fibroids cannot be detected during a pelvic exam.

What if my doctor is uncertain about what she is feeling?

She may perform further studies such as an ultrasound or CT scan of the pelvis and abdomen to help delineate the location and size of the pelvic mass. Serial ultrasound exams help to determine if a fibroid is growing over a period of time. If your doctor is still unsure, a laparoscopy examination with a direct look at the pelvic organs may be indicated to make sure the mass is a fibroid and not an enlarged ovary.

How are fibroids treated?

The treatment of fibroids depends on the symptoms they cause. The most definitive treatment is their removal by surgery. If you are still interested in having children, it may be possible to remove the fibroids, then repair the uterus to preserve childbearing ability. This major surgery is called a *myomectomy.* If you no longer wish to bear children and the fibroids are causing symptoms, a hysterectomy (removal of the uterus, but not necessarily the ovaries) is the best treatment. Occasionally small, submucous fibroids can be removed during a D & C or with a hysteroscope. Recently, laser surgery and electrosurgery through a laparoscope or hysteroscope have been used to remove smaller fibroids without major surgery. See Chapter 12 for a discussion of these procedures.

Are there any non-surgical treatments for fibroids?

Recently the use of hormones related to GnRH *(Gonadotropin-Releasing Hormone)* called analogues with either agonist or antagonist properties to GnRH have been used to suppress ovarian function and shrink fibroids. The medication most commonly used is called *leuprolide acetate* (Leupron) and is given by injection once a month. Leupron induces a menopausal state since it decreases estrogen production to levels approaching menopause. An intranasal form of a similar GnRH analogue called Synarel is also available. It is administered as a nasal spray twice a day.

If leuprolide is stopped, do the fibroids start growing again?

Yes, they do. Leuprolide causes a menopausal state and a concomitant reduction in the size of a fibroid only while it is being administered. Once the leuprolide is stopped, the fibroid's growth rebounds. This medication is often used to shrink fibroids prior to surgery. It makes the surgery easier with less risk of blood loss. If you are near menopause, leuprolide may relieve your symptoms until you reach a natural menopause, at which time the fibroids will become smaller. Leuprolide will usually relieve pain and abnormal bleeding if these are caused by the fibroids. Leupron or Synarel can also be used to shrink fibroids so a hysterectomy may be performed vaginally rather than abdominally.

What are the possible side effects of leuprolide?

Leuprolide causes symptoms similar to those of menopause. These can include hot flashes, vaginal dryness, joint pains, and a negative calcium balance with a tendency toward osteoporosis if the leuprolide is given long enough. It is usually best to take calcium while on leuprolide to keep calcium loss at a minimum. Tests are now being conducted to see if small doses of estrogen can prevent the side effects of Leupron without stimulating the growth of the fibroids.

Do all fibroids have to be treated?

Not necessarily. If a fibroid is small or is not causing symptoms it can be observed and followed to make sure it is not enlarging rapidly. You may need to visit your doctor more than once a year to keep a closer watch on its growth. Once you go through menopause, fibroids should become smaller because they are dependent on estrogen.

If I go on estrogen replacement therapy and have fibroids, will the estrogen cause my fibroids to grow?

The presence of a fibroid is not a contraindication to estrogen therapy. It is possible, however, that taking estrogen or estrogen plus progesterone may cause your fibroid to grow. Although the dose of estrogen is usually not large enough to cause a marked change, you should be followed closely as a precaution.

POLYPS

What are polyps?

A *polyp* is a growth arising from the superficial lining (*mucosa*) of an organ such as the intestine, colon, or uterus, and extending into the body of that organ. A polyp in the uterus may form either from the uterine lining (an *endometrial polyp*) or from the the endocervix, the canal leading to the uterine cavity (an *endocervical polyp*).

How do endometrial polyps form?

Polyps form in several ways within the uterus. If the uterine lining does not shed regularly or completely each month, the continual build-up of uterine lining tissue may eventually result in polyp formation. This is more common during the perimenopausal years when hormone production becomes irregular. In addition, a small piece of pregnancy tissue left after a delivery, miscarriage or abortion may become attached to the uterine lining and may not shed during subsequent menstrual cycles. This results in a *placental polyp*. A hereditary predisposition to polyps can cause certain families to have a higher incidence of these growths. (This is similar to the genetic predisposition to colon polyps.)

Do polyps ever become malignant?

It is possible but unlikely for a polyp to become malignant (cancerous) when you are in your 30's or 40's. If you stop menstruating but later develop post-menopausal bleeding, the chances of malignancy occurring in a polyp are increased. Endocervical polyps are rarely malignant.

What are the symptoms of a uterine polyp?

Persistent pre- or post-menstrual spotting is the most common symptom of an endometrial polyp. Polyps can also cause very heavy and prolonged periods. Endocervical polyps often do not cause symptoms but if they do, symptoms may include nuisance spotting or heavy bleeding.

How are polyps diagnosed?

Since endometrial polyps are located inside the uterine cavity, they cannot be seen or felt on a routine pelvic examination. Your doctor must have a feel or look inside the uterus to see if polyps are present. This is often done with an endometrial aspiration or a D & C. A hysteroscopy exam may also be performed. Chapter 12 describes these procedures.

Your doctor can usually see endocervical polyps protruding from the cervix during a pelvic exam. These are easily twisted off with an instrument.

ENDOMETRIOSIS

What is endometriosis?

Endometriosis is a disease in which the tissue that normally lines the uterine cavity (the endometrium) becomes implanted and starts to grow elsewhere in the body. The endometrial glands are most commonly found around the pelvic ligaments, in the septum between the vagina and rectum, or in the ovaries.

Can endometriosis cause abnormal periods?

The most common symptom of endometriosis is severe menstrual cramps. Often endometriosis involves the ovaries causing cysts called *endometriomas* or *chocolate cysts of the ovaries* because they are filled with dried blood resembling chocolate. Endometriomas may cause abnormal periods since they interfere with the ovaries' production of estrogen and progesterone. This condition is commonly discovered in women in their 30's during an infertility investigation, but can cause abnormal periods, ovarian cysts, and painful periods in perimenopausal women, as well.

How is endometriosis treated?

The treatment for endometriosis ranges from just observation to hormonal treatment with birth control pills or danazol to surgery. Leuprolide, a GnRH analogue has also recently

Figure 3-2

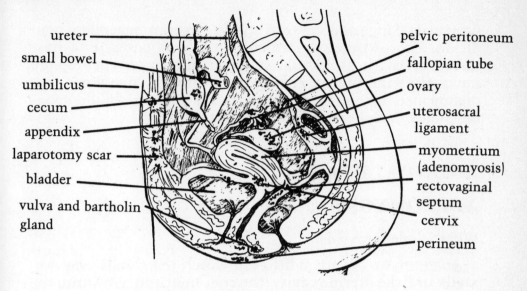

ureter
small bowel
umbilicus
cecum
appendix
laparotomy scar
bladder
vulva and bartholin gland

pelvic peritoneum
fallopian tube
ovary
uterosacral ligament
myometrium (adenomyosis)
rectovaginal septum
cervix
perineum

Various sites of endometriosis.

Figure 3-3

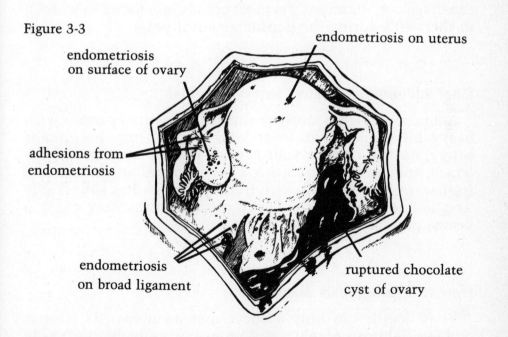

endometriosis on uterus
endometriosis on surface of ovary
adhesions from endometriosis
endometriosis on broad ligament
ruptured chocolate cyst of ovary

Uterus with endometriosis and chocolate cyst (endometrioma) that has ruptured.

been used. Since endometriosis is an estrogen-dependent condition, the ultimate treatment, in severe cases, is a hysterectomy with a bilateral salpingoophorectomy (complete removal of the uterus, tubes, and ovaries). Once you reach menopause, any endometriosis that is present should spontaneously disappear as estrogen decreases.

ADENOMYOSIS

What is adenomyosis?

Adenomyosis is a condition in which the glands that normally line the uterine cavity (the endometrium) grow into the muscle of the uterus. It is often referred to as *internal endometriosis,* since the endometrial tissue invades the body of the uterus. Adenomyosis is most commonly found in women in their 40's during the perimenopausal years.

Does adenomyosis cause any symptoms?

Adenomyosis may cause prolonged menstrual periods with heavy bleeding. Pelvic or abdominal pain may be present before, during, or after your period. The uterus may feel enlarged, soft, and tender during a pelvic exam but smooth and regular (unlike a uterus with fibroids, which has a markedly irregular feeling). The enlarged, boggy uterus may cause a heavy, pressure sensation in the pelvis.

How is adenomyosis diagnosed?

Your doctor can only suspect that adenomyosis is your problem. Unfortunately, adenomyosis cannot be positively diagnosed until after a hysterectomy when the uterus is examined under the microscope.

Figure 3-4

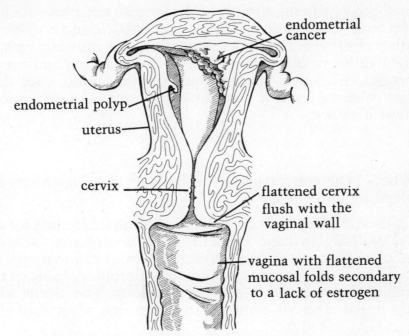

endometrial cancer

endometrial polyp

uterus

cervix

flattened cervix flush with the vaginal wall

vagina with flattened mucosal folds secondary to a lack of estrogen

Possible postmenopausal changes of the uterus and vagina.

How is adenomyosis treated?

One of the conservative medical treatments for abnormal bleeding, such as progesterone therapy or a prostaglandin inhibitors (ibuprofen) may be helpful. If your symptoms suggest adenomyosis but have not responded to these more conservative measures, a hysterectomy may be indicated.

OTHER PROBLEMS

What else can cause abnormal periods during the climacteric?

In some rare causes, abnormal periods may have nothing to do with hormonal disturbances (dysfunctional uterine bleeding) or abnormalities of the uterus. Some uncommon estrogen-producing tumors of the ovaries can cause abnormal bleeding. A disorder such as *von Willebrand's* disease or other clotting abnormality, leukemia, or metastatic cancer to the ovaries or uterus may also cause abnormal and irregular periods. Although these are not very common, your doctor may suspect them if your have other signs or symptoms of these diseases.

What if the conservative methods of treating abnormal bleeding don't help?

Often a D & C will control the abnormal bleeding for a few cycles, only to have it recur. Your doctor may suspect a problem that was missed during previous examinations, such as a small undiagnosed submucous fibroid. A hysterectomy (removal of the uterus) may be necessary. The uterus will be examined after its removal to determine what caused the excessive bleeding.

"MEDICAL" D & C

Do I need a D & C every time I have an abnormal period?

No, you don't. The decision to do a D & C, uterine aspiration, or endometrial biopsy depends on several factors including your age, the frequency and amount of your bleeding, and whether or not you have had a recent D & C. If you are between the ages of 20 and 40, and your bleeding is not extremely heavy, a "medical" D & C may be tried using progesterone therapy prior to further investigation. If you are in your 40's or 50's when the abnormal bleeding first starts, you may be advised to have an endometrial biopsy, an office aspiration, or a D & C prior to progesterone therapy to rule out the possibility of a malignancy. If you are past menopause and have not bled in the previous year and again develop bleeding, you should definitely undergo an office aspiration or a full D & C to determine the cause.

What is a medical D & C?

Essentially, a medical D & C is the same as the progesterone therapy I mentioned previously, in which one takes progesterone pills for 7 to 14 days, except that progesterone is usually given only one time rather than monthly. A medical D & C may cure abnormal periods due to hormonal disorders.

What are the advantages and disadvantages of a medical D & C?

The medical D & C is a simple treatment that may save you from undergoing a surgical procedure such as an endometrial aspiration or surgical D & C. The disadvantage of this procedure is that the doctor does not receive any tissue to analyze under the microscope for a more definitive diagnosis. If abnormal bleeding persists after a medical D & C, a surgical D & C should be performed.

4

What Are Hot Flashes?

The hot flash or flush is the most common complaint of the menopausal period. Hot flashes may cause severe anxiety and embarrassment when they occur around other people. They can even interfere with sleep. Although 75% of women have hot flashes, only 25% experience them with such severity that they seek medical attention. In this chapter, I will discuss what the hot flashes and flushes are, and what can be done for them. In addition, I will cover other common symptoms often associated with menopause such as anxiety, depression, sleep disturbances, and memory loss.

HOT FLASHES

What are hot flashes and flushes?

Hot flashes and flushes refer to the sudden onset of intense heat and perspiration during the menopausal period. If hot flashes occur at night, they are called "night sweats." The hot flash is often associated with a reddening of the skin and can be one of your most bothersome symptoms during the menopausal years.

What is the difference between a hot *flash* and a hot *flush*?

The hot flash is your own experience of the sensation, while a hot flush is the reddening of your skin observed by others. Both refer to the same symptom and are often used interchangeably depending on the origin of the writer. Americans tend to use the term hot *flashes*; the British say hot *flushes*.

Is there an actual change is skin temperature during a hot flash?

The skin temperature goes up approximately four degrees from 84°F to 90°F during a hot flash. This rise in skin temperature actually causes the body temperature to drop following the flash, as heat is lost from the skin. That's why you may feel warm but then chilled after several flashes in a row.

What parts of my body are likely to be affected by hot flashes?

Although hot flashes can occur over your entire body, the face, neck and upper body are the most common locations.

How long does a hot flash last and how many can I have over a period of time?

They may last anywhere from a few seconds to several minutes, and occasionally for up to one hour. The number of flashes experienced during a period of time varies from a few per month to 50 per day.

How long will I continue to have hot flashes?

That varies greatly from woman to woman. Hot flashes may start in the premenopausal period several years before your last menstrual period. They will often continue and may become more bothersome after the menopause. Sixty-five percent of women who have hot flashes experience them for one or two years. About 30% have them for up to five years. For a very small percentage of women, the flashes may last for up to 20 years and very occasionally, a lifetime.

Can hot flashes come and go?

Yes. It is not unusual for hot flashes to come and go over many months or even years. It is very common for hot flashes to bother you for several weeks or months, to go away for a similar period of time, and then to return. It may seem that you are going in and out of menopause.

Is there a warning before a hot flash?

Usually there is no warning, but occasionally, a palpitation or pressure feeling in the head occurs just before the flash.

THE CAUSE OF HOT FLASHES

Does anything trigger a hot flash or make it worse?

If you are prone to hot flashes, just about any change in your environment can induce them. Emotional changes such as anxiety, excitement, and fear and external forces such as exercise or change in temperature can all precipitate the sensation. Hot and spicy foods, alcohol, and caffeine can aggravate or bring them on. Hot flashes are much worse at night.

What causes hot flashes?

No one knows exactly what precipitates the hot flash. They are believed to be related to the pulsatile release of the hormones GnRH, FSH and LH from the hypothalamus and pituitary glands as the level of estrogen production decreases. This is related to a group of menopausal symptoms referred to as *vasomotor instability*.

Can conditions other than menopause cause hot flashes?

Thyrotoxicosis (an overactive thyroid gland), uncontrolled diabetes, and drug and alcohol abuse are other medical disorders in which hot flashes can occur.

Have other hormones been implicated as the cause of hot flashes?

The endocrine system is very complex and involves many different organs. The adrenal gland secretes a host of hormones including *epinephrine* and *norepinephrine* as well as *cortisol* and *aldosterone*. The interaction of all of these coupled with hormones from the hypothalamus, pituitary and thyroid glands has some effect on the vasomotor instability and hot flashes that occur during the menopausal years.

Why I am bothered with a tremendous number of hot flashes but my friends aren't?

The degree of difficulty with hot flashes varies greatly from woman to woman. Each person has an individual response to the amount of estrogen her body produces. In addition, if your ovaries abruptly cease producing estrogen (either naturally or as a result of surgical menopause), you will probably be bothered with more hot flashes more readily than a woman whose ovaries stop gradually. Many women continue to produce estrogen from sources other than their ovaries after menopause, reducing their chances of developing hot flashes.

What other organs secrete estrogen?

In premenopausal and postmenopausal women, the adrenal glands (located above each of your kidneys) manufacture and secrete male-type hormones (androgens) which the body fat converts to estrogen. This can be a significant source of estrogen production in some postmenopausal women. Generally, women who are obese will have more estrogen in their bodies during the postmenopausal years than women who are very thin.

Will obese women have a lower incidence of hot flashes?

Generally, obese women have fewer postmenopausal symptoms, such as hot flashes and osteoporosis, than thin women.

If I never had any estrogen production, will I experience hot flashes?

If you were born without functioning ovaries, such as in *gonadal dysgenesis* or Turner's syndrome, you will not experience hot flashes unless you were put on estrogen replacement therapy and the estrogen is suddenly stopped. Medical evidence indicates that hot flashes are caused by the withdrawal of estrogen, and not the total lack of estrogen.

Do men develop hot flashes?

Men usually do not develop hot flashes. Men treated with estrogen for certain illnesses (such as prostatic cancer), however, may develop hot flashes if the estrogen therapy is suddenly withdrawn. Again, this is due to the sudden absence of estrogen, even in men who usually do not have a significant level of this hormone.

OTHER COMMON MENOPAUSAL SYMPTOMS

What other common menopausal symptoms are similar to hot flashes?

Hot flashes are caused by what physicians refer to as vasomotor instability, that is, a disturbance in the vascular and nerve supply to different organs in your body. Other symptoms possibly related to the neurovascular system are palpitations, dizziness, tingling or numbness in the hands and legs, a loss of balance, altered sensory perception, insomnia, and memory loss.

What are palpitations?

A palpitation is a fluttering sensation you may feel in your heart for a few seconds to a few minutes. This irregular heart-beat is most likely related to menopause if it occurs with other menopausal symptoms. But palpitations can also result from heart disease or excessive caffeine and nicotine. If you are having frequent palpitations, stop smoking and discontinue caffeine. Many women go through an extensive cardiac evaluation only to find that all is normal and the palpitations were due to hormonal changes. Discuss these symptoms with your physician.

Could the numbness and tingling in my legs be from menopause?

Many other common ailments, such as back problems with a herniated disc, diabetes, and neurologic disorders, may cause numbness and tingling in your legs, but menopause (with its lack of estrogen) may also be a possibility. If the other medical conditions have been ruled out, a trial of estrogen may be beneficial. The very fine blood vessels which supply your nervous system contain estrogen receptors. A lack of estrogen to these receptors may cause numbness, tingling, a loss of sensory perception, and even an unsteady balance.

I am having difficulty sleeping. Can this be related to menopause?

Yes, it can. Insomnia, or the inability to sleep is second only to hot flashes as a reason women seek medical help during the menopausal years. Sleep disturbances can occur during any part of the sleep cycle: falling asleep, waking up frequently during the night, or early morning awakening. In fact, if you are experiencing sleep disturbances as well as irregular periods with an occasional hot flash, you may be approaching menopause even though you are in your late 30's or early 40's.

What causes the inability to sleep?

Several factors can account for menopausal insomnia. The actual discomfort of heat and perspiration associated with night sweats causes part of the problem. But the major factor is thought to be a dysfunction of the sleep center within the brain. The hypothalamus is the seat of the sleep center as well as the center that controls the reproductive system through the secretion of GnRH. Researchers speculate that the hypothalamus contains estrogen receptors. As estrogen production decreases during menopause, these receptors receive insufficient stimulation. Consequently, the sleep center is upset.

What can be done for sleep disturbances during menopause?

If you are a candidate for estrogen therapy, estrogen has been shown to improve sleep disturbances, along with other menopausal symptoms. If you cannot or do not wish to take estrogen, other modalities may help. Medications such as mild sedatives and "sleeping pills" may also be of benefit, but you should be careful not to become dependent on them, as you may grow immune to their effect and have to increase their dosage gradually. A well-balanced diet and exercise program help sleep patterns in perimenopausal women. Exercise stimulates norepinephrine release in the brain, which "stabilizes" the autonomic nervous system.

I've noticed my memory is slipping. Is this from menopause?

Many perimenopausal and postmenopausal women complain of memory loss. Although this appears to be a problem with all of us as we age, several studies have shown an improvement in memory with estrogen replacement therapy. Some of the memory loss may be attributed to a lack of estrogen and the menopausal syndrome. This phenomenon of memory loss in the postmenopausal woman is often referred to as the CRS syndrome—"can't remember shit!"

I've had a feeling there are insects creeping all over my skin. Am I going crazy?

This rare but strange sensation is one of the most frightening menopausal symptoms. It is called *formication* from the Latin *formica,* meaning ant. If you or your doctor are unfamiliar with this symptom, both of you may think you are going crazy. Formication is related to estrogen deprivation and can be helped with estrogen replacement therapy.

PHYCHOLOGICAL AND SOCIAL FACTORS DURING MENOPAUSE

Can I expect to go "crazy" during menopause?

The relationship between menopause and its psychological symptoms has been vigorously debated among researchers. One of the greatest myths about menopause is that women are expected to go "crazy" at this time of their lives. Although a number of perimenopausal women do experience some emotional difficulty, most sail through menopause with very few problems. The extent to which a woman experiences psychological problems depends upon a number of things, including these social factors:

- **how her cultural background regards menopause**
- **her social class**
- **whether she works inside or outside the home**
- **the degree of involvement with her children**
- **the occurrence of other undesirable life events**

The loss of close family members and a past history of psychological problems makes it harder to cope with other stresses occurring at this time.

What psychological symptoms may occur at menopause?

The psychological symptoms that have been reported to occur during menopause include:

- **anxiety**
- **tension**
- **depression**
- **irritability**
- **aggressiveness**
- **nervous exhaustion**
- **fluctuations in mood**
- **diminished energy and drive**
- **introversion**
- **intolerance of loneliness**
- **marital problems**
- **antisocial behavior patterns**
- **sense of internal frustration and inadequacy**

What is anxiety?

Anxiety is a complex emotion characterized by an underlying feeling of fear and apprehension. A person with severe anxiety looks very tense and restless. Often she shows signs of motor tension, such as the inability to sit still. She may move from one project to the next in a disorganized fashion.

Are physical symptoms present with anxiety symptoms?

Complaints such as:

- **a dry mouth**
- **sweating**
- **aches and pains in various parts of the body**
- **palpitations**
- **a rapid heartbeat**
- **difficulty breathing**
- **nausea, vomiting, and diarrhea**

may all be related to an anxiety state. Some of these symptoms may be related to medical illnesses so it will be up to your physician to decide how these apply to your specific complaint.

What is depression?

Depression is a disorder in which one's mood is persistently lowered. In addition to feelings of sadness, a person suffering from depression may also experience anxiety, loss of interest, difficulty with concentration, painful thoughts, and suicidal inclinations.

Are physical complaints associated with depression?

Over 50% of those suffering from depression experience physical complaints. These include:

- **fatigue**
- **decreased energy**
- **bodily aches and pains**
- **headaches**
- **appetite disturbance**
- **weight loss**
- **constipation**
- **difficulty breathing**
- **a dry mouth**
- **unusual feelings in the abdomen, chest, back, or head**

If I have become very nervous and depressed at the time of menopause, how can I tell if it's related to menopause or if it's from a psychological illness?

Emotional instability, increased anxiety, depression, irritability, and tension all appear to be more common around the time of menopause. Years ago, mood swings were blamed on the "change" and thought to be a normal occurrence. Today, we feel that many of these changes may be due to a decrease in estrogen. They should not be written off as "normal." If these symptoms stem from a lack of estrogen, hormone replacement therapy should relieve them within a short period of time. Severe depression is usually not attributed to estrogen deficiency and is more common in women with a past history of depression.

Can the anxiety and depression symptoms be related to psychological changes rather than a lack of estrogen?

Your anxiety, depression, irritability, and emotional swings may not all be related to menopause. You may have been home raising children all your adult life and now experience the "empty nest syndrome" as your children leave and go off to college. This change affects some women more than others. Your husband may be going through job changes and a mid-life crisis, as well. Divorce is also common during the perimenopausal years. If you have recently entered the work force, you may find new pressures from running your business or from your bosses. All of these may cause anxiety, depression, and insomnia which are similar to symptoms of menopause.

How can I tell if the anxiety and depression symptoms are related to menopause or are the result of life stresses?

It is often difficult to find the origin of these feelings. They may be caused by environmental and psychological changes and not from menopause at all. It will be up to you and your doctor to filter through these symptoms and decide what approach to take. Often it may be impossible to tell what is causing your symptoms and a trial of estrogen replacement therapy may be worthwhile to see if any of them can be alleviated in this way. Often they are. Undergoing psychological counseling at the same time may also be beneficial. In fact, a recent study showed depression to be much more common in younger women than in perimenopausal women.

Can social factors influence the psychological symptoms I experience during menopause?

Social factors are very important and can influence psychological symptoms anytime during your lifetime. Both positive and negative social factors are common during the menopausal years.

What positive social events occur during the menopausal years?

Most women view the anticipation of grandchildren, freedom from contraception and menstrual period worries, and the end to major childrearing responsibilities as positive events during the menopausal years.

What negative social events occur during the menopausal years?

The death of your spouse, parents, or children is not uncommon during these years. Deteriorating health, disability, or retirement are also events which may interrupt your life and make it more difficult for you to function.

How does my family role and working status affect the events around menopause?

If you are a typical woman, your are serving a quadruple role at this time of your life. You are acting as: spouse, mother, provider and caregiver. One of the most stressful events for parents in their 50's is the return of children to the household after a period of absence. Caring for sick parents can also be taxing.

If these events occur at the time of menopause, you may feel an added burden. If these events increase the anxiety, depression or insomnia you are experiencing, your family situation may be more responsible for your changing emotional state than menopause itself. A recent study showed that working women tolerate these stresses much better than non-working women.

Why has there been so much confusion about the psychological and social factors around the time of menopause?

Interpreting the research on the psychological and social changes a woman experiences during the menopausal years is confusing. Social scientists, psychologists and gynecologists all have had their own opinion on what might be contributing to the changes we've discussed. The symptoms of depression, tension, irritability, difficulty with concentration and memory, mood swings, exhaustion, loneliness, marital difficulty, anxiety, headaches, and inability to sleep are not uncommon during the menopausal years. Are these changes due to the changes in your hormones? Are they due to psychological swings that both men and women go through at mid-life? Are they due to social conditions? After filtering through most of the literature, researchers conclude that all of these factors—biological, psychological, and social—intermingle and play an important role in the development of these symptoms. The ideal treatment should include a psychological and social evaluation as well as hormonal treatment when indicated.

Do most women regard menopause as an unpleasant fact of life?

One of the biggest myths holds that women dread menopause. Recent data show that only 3% of women regret this time of their lives. For the majority, menopause is *not* a major factor in physical or mental health.

TREATMENT FOR HOT FLASHES AND OTHER COMPLAINTS OF MENOPAUSE

What is the best treatment for hot flashes and other menopausal symptoms?

Since the cause of hot flashes is a decrease in the production of estrogen by the ovaries, it should be obvious that the best treatment is estrogen replacement. In a healthy women who has no contraindications to estrogen therapy, estrogen replacement therapy is the most beneficial treatment for hot flashes and other vasomotor symptoms.

How should estrogen be taken?

Estrogen replacement can be given in many different ways, including orally, by injection, through skin patches, by implants under the skin, and in vaginal creams. In Chapter 13, I discuss the advantages and disadvantages of each of these various methods.

Are there other benefits to estrogen therapy?

In addition to helping hot flashes, the other vasomotor symptoms, such as anxiety, sleep disturbances, irritability, and memory loss may also be helped with estrogen therapy. Urogenital atrophy, osteoporosis, and cardiovascular disease may be prevented.

Do other medications help hot flashes?

If you cannot take estrogen, other medications such as *progestins, Clonidine, Bellegral* and androgens may be of benefit in the treatment of hot flashes, but not to the degree that estrogen would help.

What are *progestins*?

Progestins are derivatives of the hormone progesterone. If you are having regular periods, your ovaries produce progesterone after you ovulate. At the time of menopause, ovulation often stops several months or even a few years prior to your last menstrual period; therefore, in addition to a decrease in estrogen production at the time of menopause, there also is a decrease in progesterone secretion. Progestins have been shown to help hot flashes but to a lesser degree than estrogen. Although some physicians in the U.S. use progestins to treat hot flashes, their use for this purpose has not been approved by the Food and Drug Administration. The different types of progesterone preparations are discussed in Chapter 13.

What is *Clonidine*?

Clonidine is a drug prescribed chiefly for the treatment of hypertension. It has also been of some use to menopausal women who are experiencing hot flashes but cannot take estrogen. Clonidine works by binding *norepinephrine* released from the hypothalamus. Norepinephrine is a hormone that helps stabilize the vasomotor system. The sudden release of norepinephrine from the hypothalamus is one of the causes of hot flashes. The binding of norepinephrine by Clonidine has been shown to decrease hot flashes in some women. Methyldopa (Aldomet) is another antihypertensive agent that has been helpful to some women.

Who might benefit from Clonidine for the treatment of hot flashes?

As with the progestins, Clonidine is not approved in the U.S. for treating hot flashes. Some women with high blood pressure, however, who are having difficulty with hot flashes, may be good candidates. Both their hypertension and hot flashes could be treated with Clonidine. The recommended dosage is 0.1-0.2mg twice a day. Although this dosage may control hot flashes in some women, Clonidine is not as effective as estrogen therapy.

What is *Bellegral*?

Bellegral is a drug containing *ergotamine tartrate, alkaloids* of *belladonna,* and the sedative *phenobarbital.* It works by "stabilizing" the autonomic nervous system which is felt to be a source of the vasomotor instability causing hot flashes. It is usually taken twice a day in a long-acting form called Bellegral-S. If you are not a candidate for estrogen therapy or do not want to take estrogen, Bellegral may be an alternative in the treatment of hot flashes. You should not take Bellegral if you have vascular disease of your extremities, heart disease, high blood pressure or glaucoma.

What are androgens?

Androgens are hormones related to the male hormone, testosterone. Testosterone alone may control hot flashes if given in large enough doses but it may have unpleasant side effects such as hair growth, deepening of your voice, and weight gain. Androgens may also raise your blood cholesterol. If you are on androgens during menopause, your cholesterol should be monitored. The most frequent use of testosterone during menopause is a low dosage in combination with estrogen.

When is testosterone used during menopause?

Testosterone is occasionally used to treat extreme breast tenderness in women whose symptoms are not controlled by other measures. It is occasionally used in combination with estrogen if breast tenderness occurs from estrogen therapy alone or to improve the sex drive of postmenopausal women. Several groups of researchers are presently using a small dose of an injectable or oral form of estrogen-testosterone preparation for *routine* hormonal replacement therapy during menopause. They claim that women who receive testosterone in addition to the estrogen feel better, with a much higher energy level and an improved sex drive, than women on estrogen therapy alone. The injectable form of testosterone is advocated by some researchers rather than the oral to minimize side effects from testosterone first going through the liver. (See Chapter 13 regarding the *enterohepatic* circulation and the oral versus the systemic route to taking hormones.)

Do the ovaries continue to produce androgens after menopause?

Even though the ovaries stop manufacturing estrogen, the production of androgens and testosterone goes on for a longer period of time after the menopause. This may be an additional reason to use a small amount of testosterone combined with estrogen during menopause, especially in women who have had their ovaries removed (a surgical menopause).

Will the progestins, androgens, Clonidine and Bellegral help menopausal symptoms other than hot flashes?

If you are going to take medicine for the treatment of hot flashes, some of the other menopausal symptoms should be kept in mind as well as the vasomotor symptoms. Although the above mentioned medications will control hot flashes in some women, estrogen is the *only* medication that has been shown to help the entire menopausal syndrome—that of hot flashes, vaginal and urinary atrophy, osteoporosis, and cardiovascular disease. For instance, when progesterone preparations are used alone, they may help hot flashes and osteoporosis, but they may have a negative effect on the cardiovascular system. And they will not improve vaginal or urinary atrophy.

Will Vitamin E help against hot flashes?

Various vitamins and minerals have been tested for their capacity to reduce the severity of hot flashes. Among the few that have been helpful for some women is vitamin E. Dosage may be up to 1,200 units a day.

Are there other "natural" remedies that will help against hot flashes and other menopausal symptoms?

In the mid-1800s, Lydia Pinkham made a vegetable compound to cure women's "ills" during their perimenopausal years. Among the ingredients were many natural herbs that at one time were considered worthless but were later found to contain natural estrogenic substances. These include such herbs as ginseng, wild yam root, licorice root, sarsaparilla, fenugreek, *gotu kola,* and *dong quai.*

Some of these herbs may help some menopausal symptoms, but keep in mind a word of warning: By taking these herbs, you are exposed to an unpredictable amount of estrogen-like substances. Taking them is similar to taking unopposed estrogen, and these increased amounts of estrogen may cause hyperplasia, a pre-cancerous condition of your uterine lining. If you are taking these substances, you should inform your physician, as he or she may want to perform an endometrial biopsy or uterine ultrasound to evaluate the uterine lining. The influence of herbs on osteoporosis and cardiovascular disease is unknown.

Other products, such as selenium, magnesium, lecithin, and tryptophan, have been postulated for hot flashes and sleep disturbances, but they have met with little success. A well-balanced diet and moderately vigorous exercise program will probably be as helpful as the remedies mentioned above.

5

Why Is Intercourse Painful?

Your vagina and the tissues surrounding it are among the most sensitive estrogen-dependent structures in your body. From several months to several years after your last menstrual period, you may notice that intercourse becomes uncomfortable. You may feel less lubricated during sexual foreplay or penile entry. The vagina is unable to stretch, as it did previously. Intercourse may hurt to such a degree that, consciously or unconsciously, you begin to avoid it. You may also suffer from burning, itching, and recurrent vaginal infections that had never been a problem before. An unpleasant yellow or light-green vaginal discharge may develop. Occasionally, bleeding or spotting may occur.

These are symptoms of atrophic or postmenopausal vaginitis, which occurs when the vaginal tissue becomes thin and fragile.

What are the vulva?

The *vulva* are your external genitals: the *labia majora*, the hairy skin folds on each side of the opening of the vagina often referred to as the outer lips; the *labia minora*, the two thin skin folds usually concealed by the labia majora and often referred to as the inner lips; and the *mons pubis*, the area where the pubic hair grows.

The vulva protect the more sensitive tissues within the genital tract such as the clitoris and vagina. The labia majora provides a certain amount of vaginal lubrication with sexual arousal.

Are there changes to my external genital organs after menopause?

The combination of the normal aging process plus the lack of estrogen after menopause may result in a loss of pubic hair and a wrinkled appearance of the vulva. The wrinkling results from the loss of subcutaneous fat and elastic tissue below the skin. The labia become less sensitive and are less likely to swell and separate in response to sexual stimulation after several years of decreased estrogen production.

What is the function of the vagina?

The vagina is the passageway that extends from the vulva to the cervix (the neck or opening to the uterus). The vagina becomes lubricated during sexual arousal and is the organ which receives the penis during sexual intercourse. It is also the last part of the birth canal that a baby must pass through during birth.

What is the anatomy of the normal vagina?

Several layers make up the walls of the vagina: an internal mucous membrane lining, a layer of soft connective tissue, and a muscular layer. The area of soft connective tissue, referred to as the *erectile* tissue of the vagina, located between the mucous membrane and muscular layer, is made up of a large plexus of veins. It is similar to the erectile tissue in the penis. During sexual arousal, the veins in the connective tissue layer fill with blood to give the vagina a lubricated, congested feeling.

Describe the mucosa of the vagina during the menstruating years.

During your menstruating years, the mucosa of the vagina is well-lubricated and elastic (very stretchy). The surface of the vagina is thick with many folds of tissue and many layers of cells.

What happens to the vagina after menopause?

With the decrease in estrogen production, the vagina may lose its elasticity and its lubricating capabilities. The vaginal mucosal lining, which is normally several layers thick, becomes very thin, consisting of only a few layered cells. This thinness makes it prone to infections. The vagina may even ulcerate and bleed with very little contact.

Does the vagina change in size after menopause?

The vagina, normally two and a half to four inches long, elastic and stretchy, begins to gradually change when not stimulated by estrogen. The upper part constricts and becomes shorter and narrower. The cervix, which normally protrudes into the vagina also atrophies and may become flush with the vaginal wall. These changes make it almost impossible for some women to continue to have vaginal intercourse.

What are the changes that occur to the vagina after menopause called?

These changes are called *vaginal atrophy*. If the vagina becomes inflamed, infected, or ulcerated as a result of the

Figure 5-1

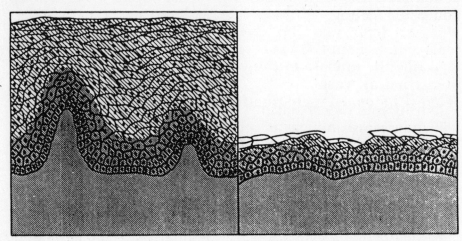

Cross section of normal vaginal mucosa.

Cross section of estrogen-deficient postmenopausal vaginal mucosa.

atrophy, the condition is referred to as *atrophic, senile,* or *postmenopausal vaginitis.*

How long does it take to develop vaginal atrophy?

As with other menopausal symptoms, the development of vaginal atrophy varies greatly. In most women, this condition usually occurs three to ten years after menopause, with an average of four to five years following the last menstrual period. Some women, however, will develop painful intercourse within three to six months of menopause, especially after a surgical menopause (when estrogen production is sharply decreased). Some women experience vaginal dryness before their last menstrual period.

Do these changes occur in all women?

The degree of difficulty you will experience depends on the levels of estrogen present in your body after your ovaries stop producing estrogen. Some women continue to have enough estrogen to prevent menopausal symptoms even though they do not menstruate. Your symptoms will have to be evaluated and treated on an individual basis. Most women, however, will eventually develop some vaginal atrophy if estrogen replacement is not started.

What if I stopped menstruating at age 38?

If menopause occurs at age 38, you may develop vaginal atrophy as early as age 40. Vaginal atrophy is related to your production of estrogen and is not a normal event which occurs with aging.

DIAGNOSING VAGINAL ATROPHY

How do I know if I am developing vaginal atrophy?

The most common symptom of vaginal atrophy is painful intercourse. *Dyspareunia* is the medical term for this condition.

How can my doctor tell if I have vaginal atrophy?

Your doctor should be able diagnose vaginal atrophy during your pelvic exam by examining your vagina. Normally the mucosa of the vagina is pink and rather thick with many folds. The atrophied vagina looks pale, thin and flattened. Lubrication is absent. If there is some question in your doctor's mind, she may perform a maturation or estrogen index.

What is a maturation or estrogen index?

Your doctor can scrape the upper third of the vaginal wall in much the same manner as she would perform a pap smear on the cervix. The cells obtained from the vagina are placed on a slide, stained with a special dye, and observed under the microscope. Three different types of vaginal cells are normally

Figure 5-2

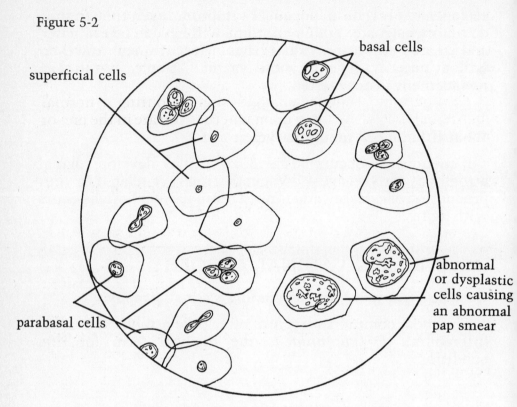

A pap smear and maturation index slide.

present: *superficial cells, parabasal cells,* and *basal cells.* The maturation or estrogen index is a set of numbers comparing these three types of cells. The greater the estrogen effect upon the vagina, the larger the proportion of superficial cells present. A total lack of estrogen is indicated by the complete absence of superficial cells. The basal cells constitute the majority of cells on the slide above.

How is the maturation index reported?

The maturation index (MI) is usually reported with three numbers such as (100-0-0) or (0-60-40). The first number refers to the basal cells; the second to the parabasal cells; and the third to the superficial cells. During the normal menstrual years, an indication of adequate estrogen production should give a reading of approximately (0-40-60). When estrogen decreases the first few years after menopause, the index will be approximately (5-90-5). A total lack of estrogen stimulation will give a reading of (100-0-0).

The maturation index changes slightly during a normal menstrual cycle depending upon whether you are in the pre- or post-ovulatory part of your cycle.

Can the maturation index be used as an indication of estrogen deficiency throughout my body?

It would be nice if doctors could perform such a simple test to determine if the other estrogen-sensitive organs are in need of estrogen replacement. Unfortunately, the maturation index only indicates the effect of estrogen on the vagina, not on other organs such as bone or the cardiovascular system. A woman's maturation index can show a good estrogen level while she still suffers from menopausal symptoms such as hot flashes. The maturation index *cannot* predict which women will develop fractures from osteoporosis.

VAGINAL BLEEDING

What is the significance of vaginal bleeding occuring after menopause?

If you develop vaginal bleeding after menopause, it is essential to determine its source. Vaginal atrophy is one of the most common causes of postmenopausal vaginal bleeding but you should not assume that the bleeding is simply coming from the vagina. Postmenopausal bleeding is an important sign of cancer of the uterine lining (endometrial cancer). Bleeding from the urinary bladder or urethra can also be confused with vaginal bleeding. Discuss all of these conditions with your doctor to determine if any further studies are necessary to pinpoint the source.

How can my doctor find the source of the bleeding?

A pelvic examination is the first step your doctor will take. To help differentiate bleeding from the bladder or vagina, a tampon can be placed in the vagina. If the bleeding continues and the tampon is free from blood, the bleeding is most likely not from the vagina or uterus, but from the bladder or rectal area. Any type of bleeding, however, has to be explained and its origin must be determined. If nothing is found during the pelvic exam, you may need an endometrial biopsy, an aspiration of your uterine cavity, or a D&C to make sure there are no abnormalities within the uterine cavity, such as polyps or an early endometrial cancer. Further studies such as a proctoscopic exam may be necessary to rule out bleeding from the rectum or a urologic evaluation to rule out bleeding from the bladder.

PREVENTION AND TREATMENT OF VAGINAL ATROPHY

Is there anything I can do to to prevent vaginal shortening and atrophy if I am presently sexually inactive?

An active sex life with vaginal intercourse is helpful in keeping the vagina well expanded to prevent shortening and atrophy during the postmenopausal years. If you are presently sexually inactive, there are several activities you can undertake to prevent atrophic changes to the vagina. Using your fingers to expand and dilate the vagina, first place one, then two, then three into the vagina. This will help keep the vagina from shortening. A water soluble lubricant such as K-Y or Surgilube will avoid trauma or irritation to the delicate tissue. This gradual expansion of the vaginal opening should be performed on a regular basis, a few times per week. Vaginal dilators are also available if you are uncomfortable using your fingers. If you are a candidate for hormonal replacement, this should also be considered.

How are vaginal atrophy and atrophic vaginitis treated with medications?

If the vagina becomes inflamed and infected because of atrophy, an antibiotic administered orally or an antibiotic vaginal cream may be used to treat the infection. An antibiotic alone, however, will not prevent the infection from recurring because the vaginal tissue will still be very thin. Estrogen is needed to thicken the vaginal mucosa so the infection will not recur. Estrogen replacement therapy is the best treatment for vaginal atrophy or atrophic vaginitis. An active sex life is also important in helping the vagina keep its shape and prevent it from shortening.

How should the estrogen be taken?

Estrogen can be prescribed in several different ways: pills administered orally, skin patch, vaginal creams, and injections. These are discussed in Chapter 13. The atrophic changes in the vagina will improve with any of these medications, if prescribed in the appropriate dosages.

What about using an estrogen vaginal cream?

An estrogen vaginal cream can be very useful in treating atrophic vaginitis. Applying this cream a few days a week can help thicken the vaginal mucosa and improve lubrication for intercourse, if that is your main concern.

You should realize, however, that estrogen applied in the vagina *does* get absorbed into the general circulation. In fact, a woman who cannot take oral estrogen because of liver disease or problems with its absorption through the intestines, can take this hormone via the vaginal route. The disadvantage of prescribing estrogen routinely in this way is its unpredictable rate of absorption into the general circulation. You really do not know how much estrogen you are getting to other organs, such as your bones.

What if I am not a candidate for estrogen therapy?

Lubricant vaginal suppositories such as Lubrin or Lubrafax or water-soluble jellies such as K-Y jelly, Surgilube, Trans-Lube and Ortho Personal Lubricant should be helpful in eliminating excessive dryness and should improve lubrication during intercourse. Two new moisturizers, Replens and Gyne-moistrin, have also proved to be helpful.

Should petroleum jelly (Vaseline™) be used as a lubricant?

It is best not to use any of the oils, perfumed creams or petroleum jellies as lubricants. These products are not water soluble and may cause excessive mechanisms present in the vagina. As a result, they make you more prone to infection even though they do help with lubrication.

If I was advised not to take estrogen, is it harmful to use a small amount of estrogen vaginal cream? Nothing else has helped my loss of vaginal lubrication.

Some doctors may prescribe a very small amount of estrogen in the form of vaginal cream to prevent atrophic vaginitis even when estrogen by other routes is not recommended. It depends on a number of factors, the most important being the original reason you were told not to take estrogen. Follow your doctor's recommendations.

6

**Why Am I Having
Urinary Problems?**

As we discussed in Chapter 5, the vagina is one of the most sensitive tissues in the body. It depends on estrogen to maintain its normal integrity and function. However, you may not realize how sensitive the urethra and bladder are to estrogen loss as well. Since the floor of the urethra and bladder are located directly on top of the vagina, they too are greatly affected by estrogen depletion after menopause. If you are in your 50's and are experiencing urinary frequency and urgency with recurrent bladder infections, you may be suffering from an undiagnosed estrogen deficiency. A trial of estrogen replacement to improve the mucosa of the urethra and bladder may be more effective in resolving your condition than the antibiotics often prescribed for "bladder infections." At the end of this chapter we will also discuss several of the pelvic relaxation syndromes such as a "fallen bladder" and a "dropped uterus," which can contribute to urinary incontinence and may be partially attributable to a lack of estrogen, as well.

SENILE URETHRAL SYNDROME

What is the urinary bladder?

The urinary bladder is a membranous sac located in the front of the pelvic cavity, on top of the vagina and cervix. The bladder acts as a reservoir for urine prior to its being expelled from the body.

Figure 6-1

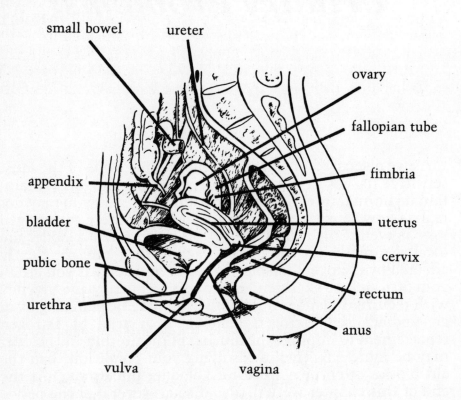

Female pelvic area.

What is the urethra?

The urethra is a one and one half-inch tube that carries urine from the bladder to the outside of the body. It runs along the top portion of the vaginal wall and empties just above the vaginal opening.

Why did I start having urinary symptoms after menopause?

The inner lining of the urethra (the *mucosa*) and the lower part of the vagina come from the same tissue: the *urogenital sinus*. This tissue contains many estrogen receptors, making it quite sensitive to estrogen. Your urethra and the bottom of your bladder (called the *trigone*) lie directly on top of the vagina and share common supporting tissues. Like the vagina, the mucosa of the urethra and bladder respond to estrogen loss and become thin and atrophic if years go by without the hormone.

What symptoms might I get if the urethra and bladder become atrophic?

Dysuria, urinary frequency and *urgency* are the most common symptoms of urinary atrophy and possible infection. The following symptoms may result:

- **dysuria: A burning sensation may occur while urinating.**
- **urinary frequency: The lower part of the bladder thins, causing a constant irritation which may make you urinate more frequently.**
- **urgency: The strong urge to urinate and the inability to hold your urine may cause you to feel that you must go to the bathroom immediately or you will wet your pants.**

If the bladder becomes inflamed, pain may also occur.

What is this condition called?

The symptoms of dysuria frequency, urgency, and pain in the bladder area in the absence of a bladder infection, are called *senile urethral syndrome, senile urethritis,* or *atrophic urethritis.* It is believed that a lack of estrogen significantly contributes to this condition.

RECURRENT BLADDER INFECTIONS

Are bladder infections more frequent during the postmenopausal years?

Unfortunately, in addition to symptoms from senile urethral syndrome, outright bladder infections can also occur more frequently during this time. The fragility of the mucosa makes it vulnerable to infection from organisms that it was able to resist during the menstruating years.

Why do I get more bladder infections than my husband?

Menopause aside, women are usually more prone to bladder infections than men because of their anatomy. In women, the distance between the external opening of the urethra and the bladder is only about one to one and a half inches long. Often, bacteria from the vagina enters the urethra and infects the bladder. Women may get bladder infections following intercourse because bacteria is introduced into the bladder during penile entry and movement. In men, the penile urethra is much longer and the chance of contamination is lower. Following menopause, the thinned mucosa of the urethra and bladder further predisposes you to frequent bladder infections.

UTERINE PROLAPSE AND PELVIC RELAXATION

Does the lack of estrogen affect any other pelvic organs?

It can. The ligaments and tissues that support the uterus and vagina may lose their tone. This can lead to *pelvic relaxation*, which includes several different conditions related to a lack of support to the pelvic organs. Pelvic relaxation can include: *uterine prolapse, cystocele, rectocele,* and *enterocele.* Any of these conditions may also be associated with urinary stress incontinence.

What is uterine prolapse?

Uterine prolapse is commonly referred to as a "fallen uterus." It is a benign condition that is not life-threatening, but can be uncomfortable. The uterus, which is normally located at the upper part of the vagina, descends into the lower part of the vagina. In the most severe cases, it protrudes from the vaginal opening. This is called a complete uterine prolapse or uterine *procedentia.*

What are the symptoms of a uterine prolapse?

The most common symptom is the sensation of a bulge at the opening of the vagina. (This may be quite frightening when first recognized, since one often associates a "lump" with malignancy.) A heavy, pressure feeling in the pelvis may also be present. Since the bladder is attached to the front of the uterus, the bladder descends with the uterus and may cause symptoms such as urinary frequency, urgency, or stress incontinence.

CYSTOCELE

What is a *cystocele*?

Cystocele is commonly referred to as a "dropped bladder." The medical term, *cyst,* is derived from the Greek word *kystis*

Figure 6-2

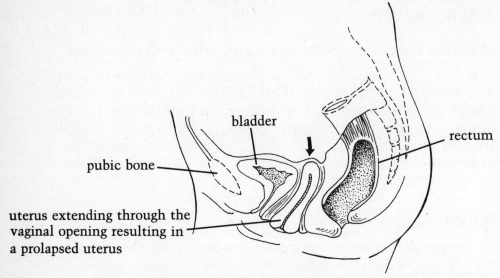

bladder

rectum

pubic bone

uterus extending through the
vaginal opening resulting in
a prolapsed uterus

Uterine Prolapse or "Fallen Uterus."

Figure 6-3

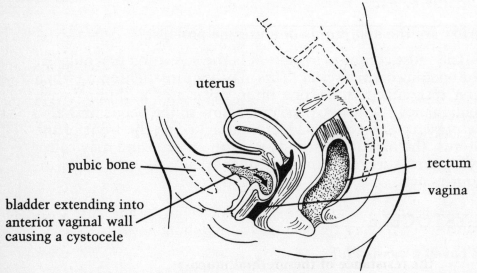

uterus

pubic bone

rectum

vagina

bladder extending into
anterior vaginal wall
causing a cystocele

Cystocele or "Dropped Bladder."

which means sac or bladder. Cystocele is a protrusion or *herniation* of the urinary bladder into the top part of the vagina when the supporting tissues between the vagina and bladder become weakened.

What are the symptoms of a cystocele?

You may experience:

- **a bulge in the vagina which may even extend outside the vagina (similar to a uterine prolapse)**
- **a sensation of heaviness and pressure in the pelvis**
- **urinary frequency and stress incontinence when the bladder doesn't empty completely**
- **a loss of the angle between the bladder and urethra**

URINARY STRESS INCONTINENCE

What is urinary stress incontinence?

Stress incontinence is an uncontrollable loss of urine associated with an increase in abdominal pressure when you cough, sneeze, laugh, jump rope, or exercise. Often stress incontinence is associated with a cystocele or *rectocele* (discussed below). In the case of a cystocele, once the normal angle between the urethra and the bladder is lost, nothing prevents the urine from dripping when pressure suddenly increases.

What causes stress incontinence?

Three factors contribute to bladder control and stress incontinence in varying degrees from woman to woman:

- **the resistance of the urethral mucosa**
- **the location of the urethra as it leaves the bladder**
- **the strength of the muscle tissue around the urethra**

The muscle fibers around the urethra constrict when abdominal pressure increases as a result of coughing or sneezing. If these muscles are weak, they are unable to constrict and urine is lost.

What is the leading cause of stress incontinence?

Childbirth causes a weakness in the vagina and its supporting tissues. The baby stretches the birth canal. As it passes through, it may tear the tissues surrounding the vagina including the bladder and rectum. The stretching of the vagina is especially common if you have had several large babies (in the 8-10 lb. range). Heredity may also predispose you to weak connective tissue between the vagina and its supporting structures. Any of the pelvic relaxation syndromes can occur (even if you have never had children) if other family members had similar symptoms.

Does the lack of estrogen contribute to stress incontinence?

Stress incontinence that occurs before menopause is usually a result of childbirth or a hereditary predisposition and *not* related to a lack of estrogen. Stress incontinence first appearing after menopause can be associated with estrogen deficiency and may resolve with hormone replacement. Estrogen will thicken the urethral mucosa, thereby improving the urethra's resistance to urine loss. It also helps the tissues around the bladder to maintain their elasticity and tone. This increased strength helps maintain the angle formed between the urethra and bladder. In addition, researchers have shown that estrogen improves the capillary blood flow and nerve supply to organs and may aid in preventing loss of bladder control previously attributed to the normal aging process.

Can loss of bladder control be prevented?

The normal aging process will eventually cause some loss of nerve supply to the bladder resulting in poor bladder control. By 80 years of age, most women (as well as men) will experience some lack of control and urine loss with an increase in intraabdominal pressure. The senile urethral syndrome, which is chiefly a result of a lack of estrogen, can be helped with estrogen replacement therapy. In some instances, estrogen therapy may be combined with dilation of the urethra. The urethra may have become scarred from lack of estrogen over a long period of time.

RECTOCELE

What is a rectocele?

A *rectocele* is the bulging of the lower rectum into the back wall of the vagina. The weakening of the tissues around the vagina that causes a cystocele also contributes to a rectocele. In this case, however, the weakness occurs between the vagina and rectum, and not the vagina and bladder, as in a cystocele.

What are the symptoms of a rectocele?

If you have this condition, you may experience:

- a bulge in the back wall of the vagina, especially during a bowel movement
- a heavy, pressure feeling in the pelvis
- difficult bowel movements which may become so problematic you have to put your fingers into the vagina and push down to force stool of the rectum

Figure 6-4

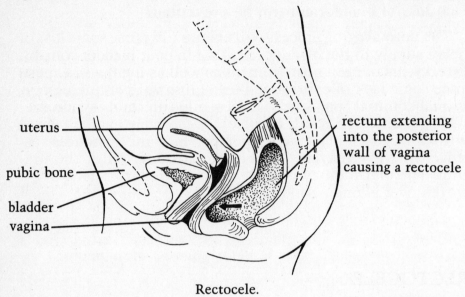

uterus

pubic bone

bladder

vagina

rectum extending
into the posterior
wall of vagina
causing a rectocele

Rectocele.

Figure 6-5

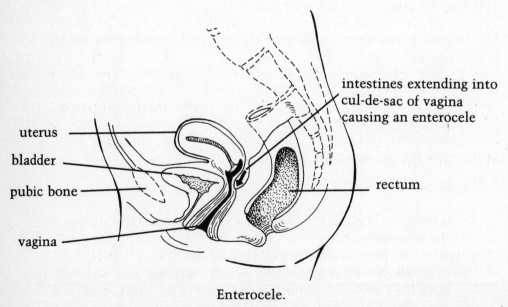

intestines extending into
cul-de-sac of vagina
causing an enterocele

uterus

bladder

pubic bone

rectum

vagina

Enterocele.

ENTEROCELE

What is an enterocele?

Enterocele, another among the pelvic relaxation syndromes, is a protrusion of the intestines through the weakened tissues between the cervix and rectum (the *cul-de-sac* of the vagina). It is often associated with a cystocele or rectocele.

What are the symptoms of an enterocele?

An enterocele cause symptoms similar to a cystocele or rectocele. You may experience a bulge protruding into the vagina associated with a pressure or heavy feeling in the pelvis. An enterocele may also occur as a complication after a vaginal hysterectomy and bladder or rectocele repair.

NON-SURGICAL TREATMENT FOR THE PELVIC RELAXATION SYNDROMES

Is the loss of estrogen responsible for the pelvic relaxation syndromes?

Estrogen loss may contribute to pelvic relaxation, but by all means it is not the sole cause. Often cystoceles, rectoceles, and uterine prolapse develop prior to menopause when your body still produces adequate estrogen. In this case, the condition is usually related to childbirth or a hereditary predisposition to weak supporting tissues. If pelvic relaxation occurs a few years after the menopause, a lack of estrogen may have contributed to the problem.

Do all cystoceles and rectoceles have to be treated?

Small cystoceles and rectoceles with or without stress incontinence do not have to be treated unless you feel your symptoms are severe enough to warrant surgery. If you suffer from complete uterine prolapse, however, it may even be impossible to walk without the uterus protruding past the vagina. This would render surgical treatment essential.

What is the treatment for uterine prolapse, cystocele, enterocele, and rectocele?

There are both non-surgical and surgical treatments for the pelvic relaxation syndromes. The degree of severity of your symptoms and your age and general medical condition will help you and your doctor decide which route you take. The most definitive and curative treatments are surgical. I discuss these in Chapter 12.

What are the non-surgical treatments for pelvic relaxation?

A trial of Kegel exercises should be the first plan of therapy. If symptoms occur prior to menopause and are not helped with Kegel exercises, surgery is the best treatment. If pelvic relaxation occurs after menopause, you may try estrogen replacement along with Kegel exercises prior to surgery. The insertion of a pessary is another approach, but this is usually unacceptable if you are still sexually active.

What are Kegel exercises?

Kegel exercises strengthen the muscle tone around the bladder and rectum. When performed correctly, they can improve mild cases of stress incontinence and the tone of the vagina. They can help tighten the entrance to the vagina if you feel "loose" during intercourse.

How are Kegel exercises performed?

Simply tighten the muscles around the vagina, bladder and anal sphincter by squeezing your vagina and buttocks and then releasing. Also, during urination, stop before your bladder is empty, then restart. You can do Kegels while sitting in a chair or at work. Several times a day, squeeze, relax, then re-squeeze these muscles, repeating at least 25-30 times during each session. It may take several months of exercises before you notice the improved tone.

What is a pessary?

A pessary is an instrument placed inside the vagina to help support the uterus, bladder, or rectum. Pessaries come in different sizes and shapes and are made of rubber, plastic, or metal. The insertion of this device is a non-surgical alternative to treating the pelvic relaxation syndromes, but it is usually unsatisfactory if you are still sexually active and mobile, as the pessary may fill the entire vagina, rendering intercourse impossible. Aside from this shortcoming, pessaries have other negative effects. They may cause an unpleasant vaginal discharge and can even erode into the vaginal wall causing ulcerations in the vagina. Occasionally, a pessary becomes so imbedded into the vaginal wall, a general anesthetic is required for removal. In addition, a pessary does not always relieve the symptoms of pelvic relaxation. Pessaries are usually inserted in elderly patients who are not good surgical candidates, since the pessary must remain in the vagina indefinitely. Once the pessary is removed, the pelvic relaxation symptoms usually recur.

7

How Long Can I
Continue To Enjoy Sex?

Years ago, the postmenopausal woman was considered a-sexual. Scientific investigation into human sexuality began only after World War I. Kinsey and his colleagues were the first to publish an extensive survey on sexual behavior. They interviewed many middle-aged and older women. These studies brought to light the fact that postmenopausal women not only continued to be sexually active, but many experienced even greater pleasure at this time, as their fear of pregnancy disappeared. Masters and Johnson's books, *Human Sexual Response* and *Human Sexual Inadequacy* further elucidated postmenopausal sexuality. We will conclude this chapter with a discussion of contraception during the perimenopausal years.

How long can I continue to have and enjoy sex?

There is no reason why enjoyable sexual relations cannot last a lifetime. If your partner is capable of intercourse, it may be continued indefinitely. You need not stop enjoying sex because of decreased lubrication and vaginal dryness. These symptoms can be cured with appropriate estrogen therapy.

What can I anticipate happening to my sex drive at menopause?

Your sex drive should not be drastically affected during the pre- or postmenopausal years. Estrogen deficiency alone will usually not interfere with your sex drive. The symptoms related to vaginal atrophy, such as painful intercourse and decreased lubrication may, however, diminish your desire for sex.

Why has my sex drive increased now that I have reached menopause?

It is not unusual to find your interest in sex *increasing* at this time. This occurs for several reasons:

- **no more worries about unwanted pregnancy**
- **more spontaneous sex with the abandonment of birth control devices**
- **no more responsibilities of raising children**
- **more time to focus on your needs and those of your spouse now**

My friend never expressed much interest in sex. She thought her sex drive would improve after menopause but it hasn't. Why not?

Some women experience decreased sex drive because they think they should, as they get older. Others never had much interest in sex to begin with. They may use menopause as an excuse to stop having sex entirely.

Now that I am ready to start enjoying sex again, my husband seems indifferent. Is this unusual?

No. Men in their mid 40's to mid 50's may experience an ebb in their sexual activity and interest because they are concerned about their ability to respond and perform. This is ironic, since the woman's desire and performance usually increase at this time.

Does it take longer to lubricate and reach orgasm after menopause?

Yes, it takes more time to respond to sexual stimulation because of many neurologic, hormonal and circulatory changes. When you were younger, the labia and vagina lubricated in a mere 15 to 30 seconds. After menopause, this process can require up to five minutes. The time needed to excite and elevate the clitoral tissue is also prolonged, but most importantly, the ability to respond remains intact.

Does it take longer for my husband to respond as well?

Yes it does. In fact, the ability to perform and maintain an erection is more of a problem for men at this age than it is for women. The recovery time (to have repeated erections and ejaculations) also becomes much longer as men age. Sperm do maintain their potency however, as men well into their 70's and 80's are still capable of fathering children.

What is the best way to deal with the difference in the sexual desire and performance between men and women at this time?

Sexual activity is more than just the physical act. Why not give yourselves more time to caress, kiss, and experiment with new methods of sexual foreplay? Communicating your desires and needs to each other as well as including more touching with your lovemaking allows plenty of time for enjoyment and gives additional response times for each of you. Intercourse is but one of may ways to express your sexual needs. If problems persist, you may wish to seek counseling.

Does a decrease in estrogen production prevent a woman from having an orgasm?

No, it does not. The ability to have an orgasm is not affected by a decrease in hormone production. In fact, some woman start having orgasms for the first time in their lives after menopause.

Does having a hysterectomy affect my ability to have an orgasm?

Although the uterus does contract when you have an orgasm, most women do not feel there is a difference in their ability to achieve an orgasm or in the quality of that orgasm if they have had their uterus removed. The vulva, vagina, and clitoris are all involved with pulsatile contractions during an orgasm and the majority of women don't miss the uterus. Some women who do notice a difference may have had some sexual difficulties before their surgery.

CAN HORMONE REPLACEMENT INCREASE SEX DRIVE?

If I start estrogen replacement therapy, will my sex drive improve?

Although estrogen alone has not been shown to markedly increase sex drive, your general sense of well-being usually improves once you start estrogen therapy, and your sex drive may heighten.

What if my sex drive is still lacking after starting estrogen therapy?

Adding a small dose of testosterone to estrogen therapy has been shown to improve the sex drive in women who have an otherwise satisfying relationship with their partners. Some researchers are using a combination estrogen-testosterone preparation, either in an injectable form once a month or in a pill taken orally. In fact, they recommend it as routine hormonal replacement for *all* postmenopausal women. These researchers claim women taking this combination feel better, experience a stronger sex drive, and have more energy than women who take estrogen alone.

Do all women produce testosterone?

Although testosterone is considered the "male" hormone, all women produce a small amount of it in their ovaries. When the ovaries stop manufacturing estrogen, testosterone levels also fall but do not disappear completely. Women who have undergone surgical menopause (bilateral oophorectomy), however, have lost their ovaries, the source of their testosterone production.

Despite estrogen replacement, some women do feel the lack of testosterone. The symptoms of testosterone deficiency in women are not well publicized but they include:

- a decreased sex drive
- a feeling of tiredness and low energy level
- a general sense of not feeling well

Adding a small dose of testosterone to the hormonal replacement regimen should help these symptoms.

Are there disadvantages to using testosterone?

Since testosterone is a male hormone, the possible side effects include:

- **a deepening of your voice**
- **excessive hair growth**
- **enlargement of the clitoris**
- **weight gain**
- **a negative effect on cholesterol and other lipids in your blood.**

These side effects have *not* occurred in most studies completed so far on the combined estrogen-testosterone treatment. The dose of testosterone is low enough to improve your energy level and sex drive without bringing on unwelcome consequences. In the future, doctors may administer small doses of testosterone with greater frequency as they gain more experience with its use. (See Table 4 for a list of estrogen-androgen preparations.)

CONTRACEPTION DURING THE PERIMENOPAUSAL YEARS

Should I be concerned with birth control at this time in my life? After all, my periods are very infrequent.

As long as you are still having periods, and you do not wish to have children, you will need birth control. Of the 27 million women in the United States in the 35-54 year old age range, 76% still have an intact uterus. Pregnancy is relatively common during the perimenopausal years. Recent surveys show 1,100 births per year in woman older than 45. Of those 1,100 live births, there were three maternal deaths each year. That's 50 times higher than the maternal death rate of women in their 20's. There were also 18,000 abortions performed per year in women over 40. All this data surely indicates a need for reliable contraception during the premenopausal years.

How long do I need to use birth control?

It is advisable that you use some form of birth control until 12 months pass without a period. At that time, you should be sterile and unable to conceive.

What types of birth control are available?

All of the methods of birth control available for the younger population are also available for you. These include condoms, foam, contraceptive sponge, suppositories, diaphragms, IUDs, oral contraceptives and permanent sterilization with either a tubal ligation for you or a vasectomy for your husband. Even though women over 40 use all of these methods, you may have additional concerns and contraindications, especially regarding the birth control pill.

What percentage of women over 40 do not use any method of birth control?

Approximately 20% of women between the ages of 40-44 *do not* use *any* method of birth control. This is a *higher* percentage than teenagers in the 15-19 year old age range and is one of the reasons there were 18,000 abortions performed on women over 40 during the last year.

SURGICAL STERILIZATION PROCEDURES

What is the most popular method of birth control in couples over 40?

Permanent sterilization either by *tubal ligation* or *vasectomy* is the most popular method of birth control in couples over 35.

What is a tubal ligation?

During a tubal ligation or tubal sterilization procedure, the Fallopian tubes are either bound (*ligated*), clamped with a rubber band, clipped, stapled, or cauterized to interrupt the tube so the sperm cannot get to the egg.

What is the most common method of tubal ligation?

Usually the physician will perform a tubal sterilization procedure by way of laparoscopy. (See chapter 12 for details on the laparoscopy procedure.) Most physicians utilize a general anesthetic in the out-patient or in-patient surgery center of a hospital. A tubal ligation can also be performed at the same time as another operation when the abdomen is opened, or it can be accomplished through the vagina or by making a small incision around the naval immediately following a vaginal birth or a Caesarean section.

What are the advantages of a sterilization procedure?

The procedure is permanent with a very low failure rate (approximately one in every 300 to 500 cases). You should be absolutely sure you do not want any more children, however, some of the procedures may be reversible but only with major surgery, no guarantee of success, and at great expense.

What are the disadvantages of a sterilization procedure?

The tubal sterilization procedure does require a general anesthetic and is minor surgery. Complications can include the risk of: bleeding, infection, and bowel injury as well as reactions to the general anesthetic. These complications are rare, but do occasionally occur. Some doctors perform sterilization procedures under a local anesthetic utilizing a small bikini-type incision in the lower abdomen called a *mini-laparotomy*. The discomfort from a mini-laparotomy is usually greater than from a laparoscopic procedure.

Are there any long-term side effects from a tubal ligation?

A small percentage of women experience cramps and irregular bleeding following a tubal ligation. This is due, in part, to a swelling which occurs in the area of the Fallopian tubes and ovaries. When a tubal ligation is performed, a small part of the *mesosalpinx*, which supplies blood to the tubes and to some extent to the ovaries, also becomes ligated. This may interfere with estrogen and progesterone production from the ovaries. As a result, irregular menstrual bleeding occurs.

If I am taking the pill and then have a tubal ligation, will my periods return immediately?

It is not unusual for menstrual periods to be "late" and irregular for several months after you stop taking the birth control pill. This is true whether or not you have had a tubal ligation. The birth control pill tends to "lighten" your periods and eliminates most of the menstrual cramps you experience. When you go off the pill, however, your periods are likely to return to their former state. Your irregular, crampy periods may return after the tubal ligation, but this is more likely the result of stopping the pill than the sterilization procedure.

What is a vasectomy?

A vasectomy is a surgical procedure in which the tube that carries sperm from the testicles to the prostatic urethra (the *vas deferens*) in the male is tied in order to prevent sperm from entering the ejaculate. After having a vasectomy, the male still ejaculates, but the ejaculate contains only seminal fluid with no sperm.

Where is a vasectomy usually performed?

If the doctor is equipped to perform minor surgery, most vasectomies take place right in his office. Many are also performed in a hospital emergency room or a one-day surgery center. Most vasectomies require local anesthesia rather than the general anesthesia that is needed for a tubal sterilization in the female.

BARRIER METHODS OF BIRTH CONTROL

What are other common methods of birth control?

Barrier methods such as condoms and diaphragm are second in popularity during the premenopausal years. Thirty percent of women this age use condoms while 10% rely on the diaphragm. The failure rate of condoms can be improved if you use it in conjunction with one of the contraceptive foams, suppositories, or sponges.

What are the advantages and disadvantages of the barrier methods of birth control?

The diaphragm, foam, suppositories, sponges, and condoms are readily available with generally low, acceptable failure rates. The foam, sponge, and suppository are more effective if a condom is used along with them.

The major disadvantage of these methods is that the interruption necessary to apply the device may exacerbate an already borderline impotence problem in some men. If the continuity of foreplay is broken, your partner may lose his erection and may not recover in time to continue to perform. For many couples, however, these methods are perfectly satisfactory.

I have been using the rhythm method of birth control with good results. Can I continue this?

As long as you have regular periods, the rhythm method should continue to be successful. Unfortunately, you will not be forewarned when your periods become irregular. Ovulation may occur at an unpredictable time resulting in an unwanted pregnancy. It is best not to rely on the rhythm method of birth control during this time of your life.

INTRAUTERINE DEVICES

Can I use an IUD for birth control?

The intrauterine device, more commonly known as the IUD, is actually one of the better methods of birth control for the perimenopausal woman if she does not have abnormal bleeding or extremely heavy or crampy periods.

On the negative side, users of IUDs suffer from a higher incidence of pelvic infections than women who do not use them. These can lead to a fertility problem which may render one sterile. Since future fertility is not a concern for most premenopausal women, this complication is not as great a deterrent as it would be to a woman in her 20's or 30's. Women with only one sexual partner have a very low infection rate, which may influence the choice of contraception.

What are the disadvantages of the IUD?

As you get closer to menopause, abnormal bleeding from either hormonal reasons or abnormalities of the uterus such as fibroids is common. If this does occur, the IUD may have to be removed as it would be impossible to determine if the cause of the abnormal bleeding is related to the IUD or other abnormalities within the uterus. An IUD may also cause more cramps with your menstrual period as well as increase an already heavy flow.

I've heard the IUD is no longer available. Is this true?

Because of the medical-legal controversy over IUDs and the many lawsuits over their use, most IUDs have been taken off the U.S. market. The Dalkon Shield, Lippies Loop, Safety-Coil, the copper IUDs, the CU-7 and Tatum-T are no longer available. At present, only two IUDs are distributed: the Progestasert and the ParaGard.

The hormone progesterone is incorporated into the stem of the Progestasert. This gives the uterine lining a progestational effect that enhances the IUD's effectiveness. This IUD is rather expensive, since it must be changed yearly. In contrast, other IUDs were good for at least three years with some doctors leaving the non-copper devices in indefinitely.

The ParaGard is a T-shaped copper IUD similar to the Tatum-T. It was recently approved for 8 years of use without having to be changed. Its popularity may depend on the legal climate surrounding its use. IUDs have become very expensive because of legal concerns. Perhaps, if only women who have completed their childbearing use IUDs, we could avoid the legal battles over their use.

BIRTH CONTROL PILLS

Can I take the birth control pill if I am over 35?

If you are over 35 and you smoke, you should not take the birth control pill. During the last several years, women between 35 and 40 and even those over 40 have been using the birth control pill more liberally. Recent data show low-dose birth control pills to be effective and safe up to age 50 in the normal, healthy female.

Why is the age range for women who can take the pill expanding?

To begin with, the pills, themselves, are becoming safer. Pills containing 20–35mcg of estrogen, considered a low dose, have become more popular over the last few years. The multiphasic pills, which reduce the progesterone dose during the cycle, are also frequently prescribed. In fact, in the fall of 1988, pharmaceutical manufacturers voluntarily removed all pills containing more than 50mcg of estrogen from the market. The reduced hormone dose should diminish the potential serious side effects from the pill, thus making them safer for women over 40. New birth control pills containing newer progestational agents which have little effect on lipid metabolism are also becoming available.

Changes in lifestyle habits have also contributed to the pill's wider use. Most women are leaner, healthier, and in better physical condition than they were several years ago. They should be better candidates to stay on the pill.

Can all women over 40 remain on the pill?

Definitely not. You must be in a low risk category. You should:

- **be of normal body weight (no obesity)**
- **have normal blood pressure**
- **be a non-smoker**
- **have a normal lipid profile (cholesterol)**

You should have no past history of:

- **cardiovascular disease**
- **blood clots**
- **estrogen-dependent cancer**

Your physician should perform a complete physical with lipid studies if you are considering continuing the pill after 40. Many doctors use 35 or 40 as the automatic cut-off for prescribing the pill. They may not even entertain the possibility of keeping you on the pill beyond that age. Recent evidence, however, confirms that if you are not at high risk, it is safe to stay on low-dose pills until menopause.

What would be the advantage of staying on the birth control pill until menopause?

Second only to sterilization, the birth control pill is a sure method of preventing unwanted pregnancy. The pill has enough hormones to prevent hot flashes, vaginal atrophy, and osteoporosis.

The cardiovascular and lipid changes that were a concern with the higher-dose pills are not a concern with the lower-dose pills. Women in their 40s who are having perimenopausal symptoms such as hot flashes, irregular periods, and sleep disturbances may benefit greatly from taking low-dose birth control pills. They not only provide adequate hormone replacement but also shut off hormone production from the ovaries. This will prevent the hormonal fluctuations causing perimenopausal symptoms. Once menopause is reached, standard postmenopausal hormones can be taken.

What is Norplant?

Norplant is a new, implantable contraceptive containing the progestational drug Levonorgestrel. It is put under the skin in the upper arm, where it slowly releases the drug over a 5-year period. Although it may cause irregular periods, spotting, and weight gain, Norplant is an alternative form of birth control for some women.

8

What Is Osteoporosis?

The bones in your body are like many of your other tissues: they are in a constant state of change. Old bone is destroyed and new bone is formed in a process called *bone remodeling*. As long as the production of new bone keeps up with the bone that is lost, your skeleton will remain strong with a low risk for fracture.

Bone loss normally accompanies aging, starting around the age of 35 or 40 in women and about a decade later in men. Prior to the age of 40, the bone remodeling process favors the rebuilding of bone that has been destroyed. The total bone mass remains stable. During the ten years before menopause, bone remodeling begins to favor bone destruction (*resorption*), first at a relatively slow rate. After menopause, bone mass decreases rapidly as bone resorption exceeds production.

Recent evidence shows that by combining adequate amounts of calcium, exercise, and estrogen you can prevent the serious consequences that result from osteoporosis.

THE FACTS ABOUT OSTEOPOROSIS
What is osteoporosis?

Osteoporosis refers to a change in the bone structure: bone loss exceeds production. The bone that remains in your body is chemically normal, but it is much thinner and can break more easily than the bone that was present previously.

Why is osteoporosis a problem?

Osteoporosis increases the likelihood of bone fractures (a break in the bony structure). In fact, it is responsible for 1.3 million fractures each year, including most of the 250,000 hip fractures that occur in postmenopausal women. The death rate (*mortality*) from hip fractures is approximately 10% to 15% higher than what we would expect in a comparable age group of women without fractures. As many as 75% of the women who suffer hip fractures lose their independence and are unable to care for themselves, with 25% of these needing skilled nursing care the rest of their lives. Approximately $10–$15 billion is spent annually on treating osteoporosis and its related complications.

How common is osteoporosis?

Studies have shown that 25% to 33% of *all* women have evidence of osteoporosis by age 60. At age 80, 25% of *all* women will have experienced a hip fracture. Twenty-five million Americans are believed to be afflicted with the disease.

How many women are in the post menopausal age?

Forty million women in the United States fall into the post menopausal age range, with half of these older than 65. Of these, one-half to one-third are afflicted with osteoporosis, therefore, a large number of women in the U.S. are suffering from the consequences of this disease.

Is osteoporosis on the increase?

It appears so, yet this is not solely related to the aging of our population. There are proportionally more hospitalizations for hip fractures in recent years than there were many years ago. The reasons for this are not fully understood.

What is the biggest risk factor for osteoporosis in women?

The loss of ovarian estrogen production that occurs at menopause is the predominant risk factor. Although bone thins with aging in both sexes, menopause is clearly the major cause for women. In fact, the earlier you experience menopause, the greater your risk for developing osteoporosis. The same is true for a surgical menopause when the ovaries are removed for medical reasons. Numerous studies have shown that estrogen replacement will prevent bone loss associated with menopause. I will discuss this and other preventative measures in more detail at the end of this chapter.

Figure 8-1

normal bone with thick bridges

osteoporotic bone with very thin, broken bridges

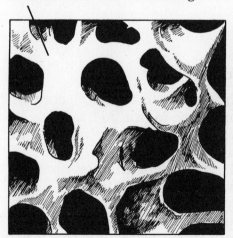
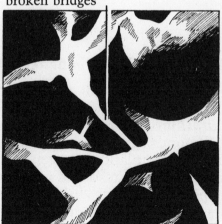

Microstructure of Normal Bone.   Microstructure of Osteoporotic Bone.

BONE REMODELING: THE CAUSE OF OSTEOPOROSIS

What is bone remodeling?

Bone remodeling is the process which enables adult bone tissue to maintain its overall composition, mass, and volume. It involves bone loss, more commonly known as bone resorption as well as new bone formation. The balance between bone resorption and bone formation is a constant, ongoing function.

How does bone remodeling occur?

Bone resorption is initiated in a small area of the bone called a *packet*. A cell (an *osteoclast*) starts the process by resorbing bone that is already present. A cavity forms where the osteoclasts have been working. Then for some unknown reason, another cell called an *osteoblast* comes in and starts forming new bone. In an ideal situation, the amount of bone that is laid down by the osteoblasts is equal to the amount of bone that is resorbed by the osteoclasts. If the new bone totals less than the bone that is resorbed, osteoporosis begins.

What controls the bone remodeling cycle?

Many factors, not all of which are fully understood, control bone remodeling. Different substances in our bodies such as *parathyroid hormone, calcitonin*, vitamin D, insulin, thyroid hormones, growth hormone, and the sex steroids such as testosterone and estrogen all have some influence on how much bone is resorbed and how much is being formed. They appear to interact with each other, either directly on the bone itself or through their influence on calcium metabolism. Bone is chiefly composed of calcium in the form of *calcium phosphate* crystals.

What determines the strength of bone?

Bones get their strength from a structure of protein fibers connected to calcium phosphate crystals. In living bones, minerals are not just stored in the bones; they are available because there is an active circulation of blood through the bone and a constant chemical interchange between bone and body fluids. When there is a reduction in the protein fibers and calcium crystals, osteoporosis occurs.

What is calcium?

Calcium is a mineral which your body needs to perform many different functions. It is essential for muscle contraction. Your heart would not beat if you had inadequate levels of calcium in your blood. Your bones contain 90% of the body's calcium. There, the calcium maintains the bones' strength while the bones serve as a calcium reservoir for the other tissues in your body.

What are the different types of bone in my body?

You have two types of bone: *trabecular* and *cortical bone*. Trabecular bone is the type found in your spinal column (the *vertebrae*). The mass or density of trabecular bone peaks around the age of 30, stabilizes for a few years, then starts decreasing. The loss of trabecular bone is dramatic during the first 5-10 years following menopause. Because of the marked loss of trabecular bone at this time, spinal column fractures are one of the first signs of postmenopausal osteoporosis.

Cortical bone is the type found in your long bones such as the arm and legs. Cortical bone mass peaks between the ages of 30-45 and slowly starts losing its mass after that. Hip fractures result from the loss of cortical bone of the neck of the upper leg bone (the *femur*).

COMMON SITES OF BONE FRACTURES

What bones am I most likely to fracture if I have osteoporosis?

There are three groups of bone more susceptible to fractures: the spinal column, the wrist bone, and hip bones. All the bones in the body, however, are vulnerable to fractures once osteoporosis is present.

What are spinal column fractures?

These are compression fractures of the vertebral spinal column. They occur in 25% of all women over 60. The average white woman who is not treated for osteoporosis will lose two and a half inches in height because of a compressed spine. If you suffer from spinal column fractures, you will eventually develop the typical "hunchback" seen in many older women.

What are wrist fractures?

Wrist fractures (*Colles'* fractures) are cracks in the area just above your wrist (the *distal forearm*). They may occur as the result of any simple fall. If you already have osteoporosis, just leaning on your wrist may be enough pressure to cause a fracture.

What are hip fractures?

A hip fracture is a crack in the part of the thigh bone that inserts into the pelvic bone (the *head of the femur*). The incidence of hip fractures increases with age in white women, going from 0.3 per 1,000 to 20 per 1,000 as women progress from 45 to 85 years of age. Eighty percent of hip fractures are associated with osteoporosis. Fractured hips in elderly women and the associated surgery necessary for treatment carry a very high complication and death rate. Some studies have shown

Figure 8-2

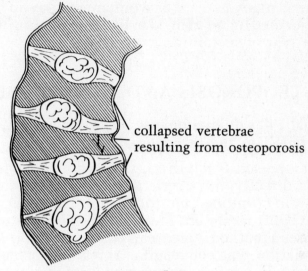

collapsed vertebrae
resulting from osteoporosis

Fractures of the spine.

Figure 8-3

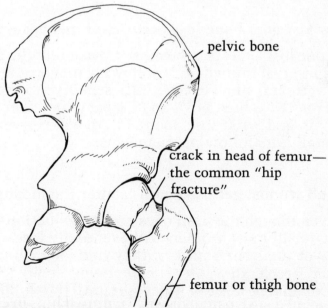

pelvic bone

crack in head of femur—
the common "hip
fracture"

femur or thigh bone

Pelvic bone and femur showing hip fracture.

that as many as 50% of women who have a hip fracture have either died or are in need of lifetime nursing home care within one year of sustaining the break.

OSTEOPOROSIS AND MENOPAUSE

What roles do menopause and estrogen play in bone metabolism and osteoporosis?

It is presently felt that estrogen does not affect bone metabolism directly, but exerts influence by interacting with *parathyroid hormone, calcitonin,* and vitamin D, three substances that control calcium metabolism. The lack or loss of estrogen causes a marked increase in bone resorption compared to bone formation. The end result is a great loss of bone in the first few years following menopause or immediately after surgical removal of the ovaries.

How fast does bone loss occur after menopause?

Bone loss appears to be most prevalent in the three to seven year interval immediately following menopause. Bone loss in the vertebral spine is especially sensitive to estrogen, where loss may be as high as 5% to 15% per year. Other bones such as the hip and wrist lose about 1% to 4% per year in the first several years following menopause.

Do all women get osteoporosis after the menopause?

Even though the level of estrogen production varies in each individual, most women will eventually lose approximately 40% of their bone mass if they live long enough. After the initial accelerated loss, the depletion stabilizes at a rate of approximately 1% to 2% per year until the woman dies. By the age of 80, most white women will suffer a 50% reduction in bone mass.

RISK FACTORS

What causes osteoporosis?

The combination of certain genetic, endocrine, and environmental factors can lead to osteoporosis. The condition is also associated with several medical disorders and therapies. Some women will be more prone to osteoporosis than others depending on how many of these factors are present.

What are the risk factors for osteoporosis?

The risk factors for osteoporosis fall into four categories:

- **genetics or heredity**
- **endocrine or hormonal factors**
- **environmental issues**
- **associated medical disorders and therapies.**

What are the hereditary factors?

The hereditary risk factors include sex, race, family history, and body build.

Are women at higher risk than men?

Women are four to five times more likely to develop osteoporosis than men of similar age. Eighty-five percent of all hip fractures occur in women; men experience only 15%.

Why are women more prone to osteoporosis than men?

Men usually have a larger body mass of bone to begin with so when they reach their 50's it takes much longer for them to thin out to the degree that it will fracture easily. In addition, men continue to produce the sex hormone testosterone well into their elderly years resulting in a slower rate of bone loss at any given age than women. Most women stop producing estrogen at the time of menopause which results in a sudden loss of bone. Both estrogen and testosterone are important in bone formation and calcium metabolism.

What influence does race have on osteoporosis?

White and Asian women have a much higher incidence of osteoporosis than black women. The latter start menopause

Figure 8-4

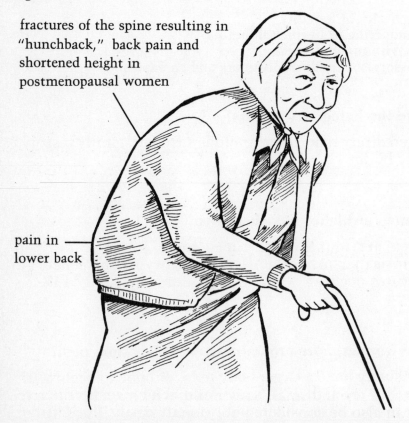

fractures of the spine resulting in "hunchback," back pain and shortened height in postmenopausal women

pain in lower back

Ramifications of untreated osteoporosis of spine.

with a much greater bone mass and must lose much more bone before osteoporosis becomes a problem. Black women also lose bone at a slower rate once they reach menopause.

What role does family history play in osteoporosis?

Bone mass and age at menopause are both partially controlled by heredity. All other factors being equal, therefore, the earlier the onset of menopause, the greater likelihood of developing osteoporosis. If your mother or grandmother suffered from thin bones, hunchback, and hip fractures, the tendency for you to encounter similar problems is much greater than would be otherwise.

How does my body build influence my susceptibility to osteoporosis?

Thin women enter menopause with much less bone and lose it at a faster rate than women of normal or large body build. Although body build could be considered in part an endocrine or hormonal factor, body fat significantly influences skeletal status, both before and after menopause. Heavier people stress their skeleton more, creating a stimulus for bone formation. In addition, the major source of estrogen in the postmenopausal women is fatty tissue. The body fat converts androgens (male type hormones) from the adrenal gland to estrogen. The more estrogen you have, the less likely you will develop osteoporosis.

What are the endocrine or hormonal risk factors for osteoporosis?

The female sex and small body build, which are hereditary factors, can also be considered hormonal issues. In addition, women who experience early menopause or who have never been pregnant run a greater risk of developing osteoporosis.

Why are women who have never had children at a higher risk for osteoporosis?

Women who have had children have a greater calcium bone mass than those who have not. In addition, childless women tend to lose bone at a faster rate after menopause than those who have experienced pregnancy. The benefit appears to come from an increased level of calcitonin (an important hormone involved with bone and calcium metabolism) during pregnancy which prevents bone resorption.

If I took the birth control pill, will I have a lower incidence of osteoporosis?

The estrogen and progesterone in the birth control pill appear to have a similar effect on osteoporosis as pregnancy. If you took the birth control pill for several years you will have a greater bone mass at the time of menopause and be less likely to develop osteoporosis.

What are the environmental risk factors associated with osteoporosis?

The environmental risk factors include:

- **nutritional risks: a lack of calcium and vitamin D**
- **excessive amounts of protein, phosphate, sodium, and caffeine**
- **a sedentary lifestyle**
- **cigarette smoking**
- **alcohol abuse**

Will calcium alone prevent osteoporosis?

Several studies have shown that if osteoporosis is already present it cannot be reversed. Calcium alone will not prevent further loss of bone but may slow down additional bone loss.

To be effective, adequate calcium intake must be combined with estrogen replacement therapy and exercise. During the first 5 years after menopause, calcium alone does not have much influence on preventing bone loss; thereafter, however, calcium is very important in preventing further bone loss.

How do alcohol and caffeine intake affect osteoporosis?

Both alcohol and caffeine accelerate bone loss in two ways. They have a toxic effect on bone and they interfere with calcium and vitamin D metabolism in the liver. The more alcohol and caffeine you consume, the greater your chances of developing osteoporosis.

How does smoking affect osteoporosis?

Smoking also influences bone loss in two ways. If you smoke, you will go through an earlier menopause, which is a high risk factor for the development of osteoporosis. Secondly, smoking appears to directly affect bone loss, even if menopause occurs at the appropriate age. Thin women smokers are extremely sensitive to bone loss. Men who smoke are also more prone to osteoporosis.

Why are excessive amounts of protein, sodium, and phosphate risk factors for osteoporosis?

A high protein diet causes an increase in calcium secretion through the kidneys. Excessive amounts of sodium and phosphate also may contribute to an increased incidence of osteoporosis by working on the complex enzyme systems of the body.

How does inadequate exercise contribute to osteoporosis?

Humans in a gravity-free state, such as astronauts circling the earth, develop osteoporosis if they stay in a weightless environment long enough. Prolonged bed rest will also result in a marked loss of bone. Adequate exercise is important in maintaining a steady bone mass, to maintain good muscle tone, and to prevent osteoporosis.

However, if other factors, such as estrogen and calcium, are absent, adequate exercise alone will not prevent osteoporosis. Exercise combined with calcium may help delay the onset of osteoporosis but will *not* totally prevent it unless estrogen is present, as well. All postmenopausal women should perform some sort of weight-bearing exercise (such as walking or running for one hour) at least three times per week to minimize the chance of developing osteoporosis.

Can excessive exercise be harmful?

Younger women who are still menstruating should be careful not to exercise to the point that their menstrual periods become very irregular or stop completely. Absent periods (*amenorrhea*) is a sign of decreased estrogen production by the ovaries resulting from extreme exercise and a lean body build. Young women marathon runners or ballet dancers who are very thin can develop stress fractures in the lower extremities from osteoporosis.

Which other medical illnesses are associated with osteoporosis?

Thyrotoxocosis (a hyperactive thyroid), *diabetes mellitus, hyperparathyroidism* (excessive production of parathyroid hormone), and *Cushing's syndrome* (excessive production of cortisone from the adrenal gland) are all associated with bone loss. In addition, women who suffer from decreased levels of estrogen production from their ovaries, and conditions such as *Turner's syndrome* (hereditary hypogonadal dysgenesis), *hyperprolactinemia,* are prone to osteoporosis if estrogen is not replaced through therapy.

Can medications cause osteoporosis?

The *glucocorticosteroids* (drugs such as cortisone and pred-nisone) may cause bone loss if used for an extended period of time. Excessive amounts of thyroid medication may also cause osteoporosis.

THE DIAGNOSIS OF OSTEOPOROSIS

What are the symptoms of osteoporosis?

Until you fracture a bone, you may be unaware that you have osteoporosis. Often, there are no symptoms. A backache in the mid- to upper back may be the first sign of the condition. This may indicate a compression fracture of one of the vertebrae in the spine.

How is osteoporosis diagnosed?

Osteoporosis is diagnosed by measuring bone density. With the increased concern about osteoporosis during the last several years, new technologies are developing fast to measure bone loss. Presently, most physicians feel that dual energy X-ray absorptiometry (DXA) is the most reliable method. There is very little X-ray exposure, and bone loss in the spine and hip can be measured with great accuracy.

Can the standard X-ray of the wrist or spine detect early osteoporosis?

The standard X-ray cannot diagnose osteoporosis until ap-proximately 30% of the bone is already lost. Therefore it is not helpful in detecting early osteoporosis. The standard X-ray machine is, however, utilized in a technique called radiographic absorptiometry (RA). An X-ray is taken of the hand next to a calibrated piece of metal of known density. The X-ray is then sent to a central laboratory where it is analyzed and the bone density determined. This technique may gain popularity as it makes bone density measurements available without expensive machinery. Other methods of determining bone density include single- and dual-photon absorptiometry and CT scanning.

What is single-photon absorptiometry?

This is a technique developed several years ago which utilizes a low-energy *radioisotope* to measure the penetration of photons through bone. The thicker the bone, the greater number of photons it will absorb. This test is usually performed on the wrist but cannot be used to measure the hip bone or the spine because of the other soft tissues surrounding the bones in those areas. The amount of radiation exposure with this technique is about 5 mrem. (A standard chest X-ray study exposes a person to 30 to 60 mrem.)

What is dual-photon absorptiometry?

Dual-photon absortiometry is a technique that uses the isotope *gadolinium-153* which emits photons of two different energies. This allows for the penetration into larger body masses to examine the spine or hip. The radiation dose of this technique is also low, with 5 to 15 mrem exposure.

What is a CT scan?

The CT *(computerized axial tomography)* scan can be used to determine bone density. A scan is taken through the backbone (the *vertebral bodies* in the spine). Its thickness is computed and compared with that of other people in the same age range. The reading tells what percentage of bone loss has occurred relative to the general population. The CT scan is used to measure bone density in the spine but not in the hip or wrist. The radiation with a CT scan is higher than in absorptiometry, with about 200 mrem of exposure.

Can the amount of calcium I lose in my urine be measured?

The calcium that you excrete in your urine can be measured by obtaining a 24-hour urine collection. This figure is compared to the amount of *creatinine* you lose. Creatinine is a product of body metabolism. Its excretion is constant in most people. A calcium/creatinine ratio greater than 0.4 is considered high and may indicate that you are losing excess calcium and developing osteoporosis. Another substance in the urine called *hydroxyproline*, a major protein in bone, has also been used to determine if excessive bone loss is occurring. Recently, measuring urinary collagen cross-links has been shown to be a sensitive index of bone resorption.

How accurate are the above radiologic and urine studies?

The newer methods of bone density measurements are fairly accurate. Their value may lie more in following measurements of several bone densities over a period of time rather than a single measurement.

Should I have one of the X-ray studies to determine if I am developing osteoporosis?

It is probably unwarranted to screen all postmenopausal women for osteoporosis. If you are in a "high risk" category, however, you should be screened. This will depend on how your doctor utilizes these techniques, as their use is controversial among experts. If you are experiencing other menopausal symptoms, such as hot flashes and vaginal dryness, estrogen therapy will be indicated with the prevention of osteoporosis as an important secondary benefit. The tests I've mentioned may be indicated only if you are being evaluated for estrogen replacement therapy for the sole purpose of preventing this disease or in evaluating the response to treatment in someone with osteoporosis.

ESTROGEN REPLACEMENT AND THE TREATMENT OF OSTEOPOROSIS

Can osteoporosis be prevented?

The prevention of osteoporosis must take a multipronged approach. Your first steps will be correcting high-risk factors by consuming adequate calcium and getting plenty of exercise. Avoid cigarette smoking, alcohol abuse, and caffeine. If you are not producing estrogen in the postmenopausal period, you should consider estrogen replacement therapy. Imagine a three-legged stool, with estrogen, calcium, and exercise each representing a leg: if one leg is taken away, the stool falls.

What medication has been most useful in preventing osteoporosis?

After numerous studies performed over the last several years on thousands of women, estrogen therapy has emerged as the single most useful agent in preventing postmenopausal osteoporosis.

How does estrogen prevent bone loss?

No one knows exactly how estrogen is incorporated in bone metabolism. It is believed that estrogen helps stimulate the production of the hormone calcitonin and interacts with two other substances, parathyroid hormone and Vitamin D which influence calcium and bone metabolism. Estrogen does *not* appear to act on the bone directly.

How much estrogen do I need to prevent osteoporosis?

The estrogen equivalent of 0.625mg of conjugated estrogen (Premarin) is the minimal amount that has been shown to prevent osteoporosis. Recent studies also indicate that combining a calcium intake of 1500mg per day, a good exercise program, and 0.3mg of conjugated estrogen (Premarin) may also be sufficient. Equivalent doses of other estrogen medications, such as Ogen (0.625mg), the Estraderm patch (0.05mg), and Estrace (1mg), are equally effective.

How long must I take estrogen to prevent osteoporosis?

The greatest degree of bone loss occurs during the several years immediately following menopause. If estrogen replacement is started for the prevention of osteoporosis, it should be taken for at least seven to ten years after menopause. As you can see, the prevention of osteoporosis with estrogen is a long-term proposition. As long as you take adequate doses of estrogen and calcium and get enough exercise, you should be able to prevent osteoporosis. As soon as you stop taking estrogen, however, the benefit ceases, but you will still be further ahead than if you had never been on estrogen replacement therapy.

Is it ever too late to start estrogen replacement therapy?

No, it is not. If osteoporosis is not found until you are 70 or 80, you can still start estrogen replacement therapy, as long as there are no contraindications. Estrogen replacement therapy will not replace bone that is already lost, but it should help prevent further bone loss.

OTHER MEDICAL TREATMENTS FOR OSTEOPOROSIS

What other modalities and medications have been used in treating and preventing osteoporosis?

Although estrogen therapy is the treatment of choice in the postmenopausal woman, not all women can take it. Women with estrogen-dependent cancer of the breast, for example, must seek out other modalities. Progestins alone, anabolic steroids, calcium, vitamin D, calcitonin, parathyroid hormone, and exercise have all been incorporated in regimens to prevent osteoporosis. A new class of drugs called bisphosphonates has recently been shown to prevent bone loss and reduce the risk of fracture.

What are progestins?

Progestins are hormones related to progesterone which are produced by the corpus luteum of the ovary after a woman ovulates. (See Chapter 2.) It is normally present in your body during your menstrual years.

Do progestins help prevent osteoporosis, as well?

Several studies have shown that progestins used either alone or in combination with estrogen will help prevent bone loss and can possibly even stimulate new bone formation.

What is etidronate?

Etidronate (Didrone) belongs to a new class of drugs called bisphosphonates, which have been shown to be effective in preventing bone loss. Etidronate is usually taken cyclically for two weeks every three months. The drug is presently waiting for FDA approval as a preventative treatment for bone loss. Several other bisphosphonates are also in the investigational stages.

What are anabolic steroids?

Anabolic steroids are hormones related to testosterone. If they are withdrawn from men (as in castration for treatment of prostatic cancer), osteoporosis will usually develop.

Can anabolic steroids be used to treat women with osteoporosis?

Studies in women have shown that anabolic steroids will prevent bone loss and increase total body calcium in women. However, their use in postmenopausal osteoporosis will be limited because of the side effects related to the male hormone, testosterone, including weight gain, hair growth, deepening of the voice, and a negative effect on the cholesterol and lipids in the body. A small dose of testosterone is being used in combination with estrogen for hormonal treatment in some postmenopausal women, without bothersome side effects.

If I have osteoporosis, is it possible to replace the bone I already lost?

As a general rule, the usual treatments for osteoporosis—estrogen, calcium, and exercise—help prevent further bone loss, but they do not replace the majority of bone you have already lost. Once osteoporosis is present, it is very difficult to replace the lost bone. Recent data, however, show that estrogen and calcitonin can increase bone density slightly, but not totally replace lost bone.

What is calcitonin?

Discovered in the early 1960s, calcitonin is a hormone produced by the thyroid gland. Although the exact mechanism of calcitonin's action is unknown, it has been shown to inhibit bone resorption and is crucial for bone metabolism. Calcitonin inhibits the activity of the osteoclast, the cell that resorbs bone. In 1984, calcitonin was shown to be highly beneficial in replacing bone mass that had already been lost. It has been theorized that exercise causes a release of calcitonin which prevents resorption of bone and osteoporosis.

Who might benefit from calcitonin therapy?

Calcitonin is presently available only by injection. A nasal spray containing calcitonin is awaiting FDA approval. Patients can learn to give themselves injections, just as diabetics can administer their own insulin.

A good candidate for calcitonin therapy is a young woman with breast cancer in whom ovarian failure has developed either from chemotherapy or surgical removal of her ovaries. In her case, estrogen replacement is contraindicated because her tumor was estrogen-dependent. Otherwise, estrogen is still considered the recommended medication for the prevention of osteoporosis if there are no contraindications to its use.

Will exercise alone prevent osteoporosis?

Several studies have suggested that simple exercise can influence and possibly increase bone mass, but only with proper calcium intake and in the presence of estrogen. Walking and running exercises for as little as one hour, two to three times a week increases the bone mass of the spine and bones of the extremities. It has still not been established that exercise alone will totally prevent osteoporosis, especially without estrogen replacement. Extreme exercise to the point of causing amenorrhea (absent periods) in women should be avoided as this will decrease estrogen production by the ovaries and may actually cause osteoporosis.

CALCIUM AND THE PREVENTION OF OSTEOPOROSIS

Will calcium alone prevent osteoporosis?

The normal recommended dietary intake of calcium of 1000mg per day will not prevent osteoporosis in the postmenopausal woman. In fact, calcium without estrogen—no matter how much is given—will not prevent bone loss in the spinal column (trabecular bone). Calcium in the amount of 1500mg per day has been shown to be of some benefit in preventing bone loss in the extremities (cortical bone), thus reducing the incidence of hip fractures. If you are on estrogen therapy, smaller amounts of estrogen may be required if an adequate calcium intake is present.

Will calcium and exercise alone prevent bone loss?

Calcium and exercise may slow the rate of bone loss, but will not totally prevent it. Estrogen therapy when combined with adequate calcium and exercise is the only medication that has been shown to totally prevent osteoporosis.

How much calcium is needed?

The recommended dietary allowance (RDA) of calcium is 1000mg per day for the average adult. Various studies have shown that the average intake of calcium in most women is about 400–500mg per day. This falls far short of the conservative recommended dosage. It is no wonder that most adults are in a negative calcium balance with a tendency to develop osteoporosis. The current recommendation for postmenopausal women is 1500mg of calcium per day to prevent osteoporosis. Premenopausal women should try to be on at least 1000mg of calcium per day. Vitamin D is also needed as it helps absorb calcium from the intestinal tract.

What are the best sources of calcium?

Dairy products such as yogurt, cheeses, and milk are the best dietary sources of calcium. They contain significant levels of calcium in a highly absorbable form: 80% to 90% of the calcium in milk products is absorbed by the body. Sardines and canned salmon are also good sources of both protein and calcium. Most fruits, vegetables, and grains are not good sources of calcium (except dark green vegetables) and may contain substances such as fiber and oxalic acid which tend to interfere with calcium absorption from the intestines. (See Table 1 on page 140 for the calcium levels in certain foods.)

Do I need calcium supplements?

It is usually very difficult to obtain 1500mg of calcium from dietary intake alone, unless you eat or drink a lot of dairy products. Therefore, it is best to supplement your diet with one of the calcium preparations in a dose of 500mg to 1000mg per day depending on your diet.

When is it best to take calcium?

Calcium is best absorbed when ingested in small amounts throughout the day. The following types of food interfere with calcium absorption and should be avoided within two hours of taking calcium: excessive fiber (more than 30g/day); oxalates (found in spinach, beets, parsley, rhubarb, squash, tea, and coffee); phytates (found in legumes); aluminum (found in some antacids); and caffeine (found in chocolate, tea, coffee, and sodas).

I've heard that *Tums*™ is a good source of calcium. Is this true?

Each *Tums*™ tablet contains 200mg of calcium carbonate. Taking *Tums*™ is one way of supplementing your diet with calcium. Other good sources of calcium are *Caltrate 600*™ and *OsCal 500*™, containing 600mg and 500mg of calcium respectively. Numerous other calcium preparations are available, some of which are better tolerated than others. (See Table 2 on page 141.) A new, effervescent form of calcium citrate marketed as NutraVescent seems to be very well tolerated and well absorbed.

Are there side effects to calcium?

The most common complication of excess calcium is the development of calcium kidney stones, but these are rare if supplemental calcium is no greater than 1000mg per day and total calcium intake does not exceed 1500mg. Certain calcium preparations may also cause abdominal discomfort and a feeling of gassiness. You may have to try several different calcium preparations before finding one that you tolerate well.

What's the best way to prevent osteoporosis?

Here are my recommendations:

- **avoid the lifestyle factors of alcohol, caffeine, and smoking**
- **eat healthy foods with an adequate calcium intake**
- **supplement your diet to include 1500mg of calcium per day**
- **follow a planned weight-bearing exercise program at least two to three times a week**
- **take estrogen if you are not producing your own after menopause**

TABLE 1			
CALCIUM CONTENT OF FOODS			
TYPE OF FOOD	AMOUNT OF FOOD	MG OF CALCIUM	CALORIES
Dairy			
Yogurt, low fat plain	1 c.	415	145
Skim ricotta cheese	1/2 c.	335	170
Low-fat milk (2%)	1 c.	300	120
Soft-serve ice cream	1/2 c.	275	110
Vanilla ice cream	1/2 c.	100	140
Swiss cheese	1 oz.	270	105
Cheddar cheese	1 oz.	210	110
American cheese	1 oz.	175	105
Low-fat cottage cheese	1/2 c.	75	90
Protein			
Sardines with bones	3 oz.	370	170
Salmon with bones, canned	3 oz.	165	105
Chicken	3 oz.	10	140
Tuna	3 oz.	5	110
Hamburger patty	3 oz.	10	225
Egg	1 lg.	30	90
Combination Foods			
Cheese pizza (14 in)	1/4 slice	330	450
Macaroni with cheese	1/2 c.	180	220
Taco with cheese	1	175	190
Fruits and Vegetables			
Spinach	1/2 c.	85	20
Broccoli	1/2 c.	70	25
Green beans	1/2 c.	30	15
Orange	1 med.	55	70
Apple	1 med.	10	85
Grains			
Whole wheat bread	1 slice	20	70
Cooked spaghetti	1 c.	15	215
Cooked rice	1/2 c.	10	80

TABLE 2		
CALCIUM CONTENT OF SUPPLEMENTS		
BRAND NAME	TYPE OF CALCIUM	AMOUNT OF ELEMENTAL CALCIUM
Calcet	Calcium Carbonate Calcium Gluconate Calcium Lactate	152.8mg
Caltrate 600™	Calcium Carbonate	600mg
Caltrate Jr.™ (chewable)	Calcium Carbonate	300mg
NutraVescent	Calcium Citrate	500mg
OsCal 500™	Calcium Carbonate	500mg
OsCal 250™	Calcium Carbonate	250mg
Posture™	Calcium Phosphate	600mg
Tums™ (antacid)	Calcium Carbonate	200mg
Generic	Calcium Lactate	100mg
Generic	Calcium Gluconate	47 or 62mg

9

How Does Menopause Affect My Heart and Vascular System?

Cardiovascular disease is the leading cause of death in the United States. Approximately 650,000 men and women die from heart attacks and strokes every year. Before the age of 50, the risk of having a heart attack is six to seven times greater for a man than for a woman. Beyond the age of 60, the risk appears to even out. In this chapter, I will discuss why the incidence of cardiovascular disease rises after menopause and what can be done to reverse the trend to the premenopausal period. I also cover some nutritional aspects related to cardiovascular disease.

CARDIOVASCULAR DISEASES

What are cardiovascular diseases?

Cardiovascular diseases strike the heart and blood vessels. The two major kinds of cardiovascular disease are strokes and coronary artery disease. The latter is most prevalent in post-menopausal women.

What is coronary artery disease?

Coronary artery disease is caused by *atherosclerosis,* a condition that decreases the blood supply to the heart muscle. The narrowing and blockage of the coronary arteries deprive the heart muscle of adequate oxygen-rich blood and nutrients. This may damage the heart muscle, leading to chest pain, heart attack, and death.

What are the coronary arteries?

These blood vessels supply oxygen and nutrients directly to the heart muscle. They originate from the aorta just as it leaves the heart. The two principal coronary arteries, the right coronary and left coronary, divide into many small branches eventually supplying the entire heart muscle with nutrients and oxygen.

What is a heart attack?

A heart attack is the common name for blockage of one of the branches of the coronary arteries causing the heart muscle supplied by that artery to die or *infarct.* The medical name for a heart attack is a *myocardial infarction.* The area of the heart muscle supplied by the blocked artery actually dies and becomes scarred if a heart attack occurs.

What is *angina pectoris*?

Angina pectoris is chest pain caused by an insufficient amount of nutrients and oxygen reaching the heart muscle because of a narrowing of one of the coronary arteries or its branches. Another name for this condition is *coronary insufficiency.* Angina can be considered a warning symptom to a pending heart attack.

Figure 9-1

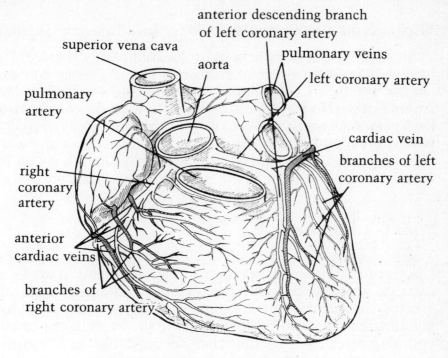

anterior descending branch
of left coronary artery

superior vena cava

pulmonary veins

aorta

left coronary artery

pulmonary
artery

cardiac vein

branches of left
coronary artery

right
coronary
artery

anterior
cardiac veins

branches of
right coronary artery

Blood supply to the heart showing the coronary
artery and veins.

Figure 9-2

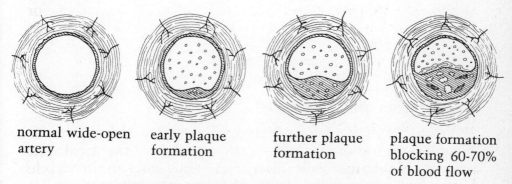

normal wide-open
artery

early plaque
formation

further plaque
formation

plaque formation
blocking 60-70%
of blood flow

Cross section of coronary artery showing
progression of plaque formation leading to
occlusion—the end result of coronary artery
disease.

What are the symptoms of coronary insufficiency (angina)?

A crushing chest pain usually located below the *sternum* (breast bone) that occurs on exertion is the most common angina symptom. The pain may radiate into the left arm. Angina may also feel like heartburn. In fact, it is not unusual for a person to try antacids to relieve the pain. Occasionally, a person may get a sudden, fatal heart attack without any warning symptoms. If you are having any symptoms that you feel may be related to your heart, see your physician promptly.

What is *atherosclerosis*?

Atherosclerosis is a type of "hardening of the arteries." Cholesterol, fat, and other blood components build up on the interior walls of the blood vessels. As atherosclerosis progresses, the coronary arteries narrow so that oxygen-rich blood and nutrients have difficulty reaching the heart. If one of your coronary arteries or its branches becomes blocked, you may have a heart attack. If the blockage is partial, you may experience the chest pain characteristic of angina pectoris. Atherosclerosis can also affect other arteries, causing a stroke if the narrowing occurs in blood vessels that supply the brain or pain in your legs during exercise (*claudication*) if the major arteries to the lower extremities are blocked. (See illustration on page 145.)

What causes atherosclerosis?

Deposits of cholesterol and other fatty substances, or plaques, on the inner walls of the arteries are the most common cause of atherosclerosis. These start early in life in both sexes, but men develop them at a faster rate than women. The plaques may build up slowly, eventually blocking (*occluding*) the coronary arteries and causing either angina or a heart attack.

What is a stroke?

A stroke is the common name for a blockage or rupture of one of the arteries that supplies nutrients and oxygen to the brain. If the main artery in the neck (*carotid arteries*) becomes blocked, a major stroke could develop due to the brain being deprived of oxygen. If one or several of the smaller arteries become blocked, a series of smaller strokes can occur. Atherosclerosis is a major contributor to strokes.

What are the symptoms of a stroke?

These vary depending on which artery in the brain becomes occluded. For example, if the blockage occurs in an artery of that brain that:

- **controls movement in your hand, you could have weakness of your grip**
- **controls your balance, you could be unsteady on your feet**
- **controls your speech, you could have slurred speech**

A major stroke can also occur by a sudden hemorrhage into the brain or a total occlusion of a major artery. Both of these can cause sudden death.

MORTALITY RATES

How do death rates from cardiovascular disease in women compare with those of men?

Death from heart attacks is much lower in young women than it is in young men. Heart attack mortality rises in both groups with increasing age, but the rate of the rise is greater for women than men. Young women and men have about the same death rate from strokes; however, with increasing age, stroke mortality for men exceeds that for women.

Has the mortality from cardiovascular disease changed in the last 20 years?

Death from heart attacks and strokes has decreased approximately 30% during the last 20 years time.

What is the reason for this decrease?

The decline in heart attack mortality has been attributed to improved medical care and changes in lifestyle. Cigarette smoking has decreased by 26% in men and 8% in women during recent years. More attention has also been given to physical fitness, weight control, and low cholesterol diets, all of which are helpful in preventing atherosclerosis. The marked reduction in heart attacks in women corresponds to the increased use of estrogen.

THE RISK FACTORS

What is a risk factor?

A risk factor is a habit, trait, or condition in a person that is associated with an increased chance of developing a disease.

What are the major risk factors for atherosclerosis and coronary heart disease?

- high blood pressure
- cigarette smoking
- family history of coronary artery disease before age 55
- diabetes
- vascular disease secondary to other medical disorders
- obesity
- male sex
- menopause without estrogen replacement therapy

What is the major risk factor for the development of strokes?

High blood pressure appears to be the major risk factor for stroke and coronary heart disease, alike. Menopause does *not* appear to be a risk factor for the development of a stroke.

CHOLESTEROL AND CARDIOVASCULAR DISEASE

What are lipids?

Lipids are the fatty substances in our blood and body tissues. *Cholesterol* and *triglycerides* are the most commonly known lipids. High cholesterol is believed to be one of the most important risk factors in the development of atherosclerosis and coronary heart disease. Although it is less clear, an elevated triglyceride level may also be associated with a higher risk for cardiovascular disease, especially if it is associated with a high cholesterol.

What is cholesterol?

Cholesterol is a soft, waxy, fatty substance *needed* for normal body function. It is used in the manufacture of hormones, bile acid, and vitamin D and is present in all parts of the body including the nervous system, muscle, skin, liver, intestines, heart, and most other organs. A high level of blood cholesterol leads to an increased incidence of atherosclerosis and coronary artery disease.

What are lipoproteins?

Lipoproteins are protein-coated packages that carry fat and cholesterol through the blood, delivering them where they are needed. Cholesterol attaches to these proteins so it can be transported to the various organs of the body.

How are lipoproteins classified?

Lipoproteins are classified according to their density. There are two types in your blood: *High density lipoproteins* (HDL) and *low density lipoproteins* (LDL). Although recent research has shown that these can be further subdivided, it is easier to understand the influence of the lipoproteins on coronary artery disease by simply referring to these two categories.

What are the HDL?

High density lipoproteins (commonly referred to as HDL-cholesterol) contain only a small fraction of the total cholesterol in your body. They carry cholesterol *away* from cells and tissues to the liver for *excretion.* For that reason, HDL is often called the "good cholesterol." It is best to have a high level of HDL-cholesterol due to its positive role in cholesterol excretion. *Low levels of HDL* are associated with an *increased* risk for the development of coronary artery disease.

What are the LDL?

The low density lipoproteins contain the largest concentration of cholesterol in your blood. LDL is responsible for delivering cholesterol to the various organs and depositing cholesterol in the artery walls. *High levels of LDL* are associated with an *increased* risk for the development of coronary artery disease. LDL is often referred to as the "bad cholesterol."

Am I better off having a high or low level of HDL and LDL cholesterol?

It is better if you have a low LDL-cholesterol ("bad") and a high HDL-cholesterol ("good").

What are the normal ranges of blood cholesterol?

The following blood levels of total, LDL, and HDL cholesterol are presently considered normal. Of you have a higher than normal range for the total and LDL-cholesterol you will run a greater risk for developing coronary artery disease.

	DESIRABLE	BORDERLINE-HIGH RISK	HIGH RISK
Total cholesterol	less than 200mg/dl	200–239mg/dl	greater than 240mg/dl
LDL-cholesterol	less than 130mg/dl	130–159mg/dl	greater than 160mg/dl
HDL-cholesterol	greater than 55mg/dl	35–55mg/dl	less than 35mg/dl

Your total cholesterol divided by your HDL cholesterol should be 4.5 or less. Anything greater than 4.5 carries a higher risk of cardiovascular disease.

What affects my level of blood cholesterol?

The cholesterol in your blood comes from two sources: what your body produces and what you eat. *The cholesterol that your body produces is all that your body needs to function.* The cholesterol you get in your diet only serves to increase your blood cholesterol level. Your cholesterol profile is determined largely by genes you inherited from your parents, but it can be strongly influenced by your diet.

What should I do if I have high cholesterol?

See your physician for a complete physical, including blood test. If your initial screening shows cholesterol in the high risk range, you should have your HDL and LDL cholesterol checked. If your total cholesterol is normal, these additional test are unnecessary. But have your total cholesterol rechecked every few years during physical exams, as a precaution. If your total cholesterol falls on a borderline-high risk or high risk range, you should follow a low cholesterol diet, and if you are overweight, reduce to your ideal weight. If you have not succeeded in lowering your cholesterol level after several months of dieting, cholesterol-lowering medications are available but should be taken only under your physician's supervision and in conjunction with a low cholesterol diet. Remember, the higher your cholesterol, the greater your risk of developing coronary artery disease. In fact, a recent study showed that for every 1% reduction in cholesterol, you reduce the risk of heart attack by 2%.

CHOLESTEROL AND THE FOODS YOU EAT

What are the basic food nutrients and how many calories do they provide?

Three basic food nutrients supply calories to the body:

- **fat provides 9 calories per gram (454 grams = 1 lb.)**
- **protein provides 4 calories per gram**
- **carbohydrates provide 4 calories per gram**

What are the different types of fat in our diet?

There are two types of fat: *saturated* and *unsaturated*. Saturated fats are chiefly found in animal products such as meat, poultry, and whole milk dairy products including butter, cream, milk, and ice cream. Some vegetable oils like coconut, palm kernel, and palm oils also contain saturated fats. These fats raise blood cholesterol more than anything else in your diet and should be avoided if you have a high or borderline-high cholesterol.

What are the unsaturated fats?

The unsaturated fats are usually liquid at room temperature. There are two types of unsaturated fats: *monounsaturated* and *polyunsaturated*. The monounsaturated fats are found in foods that come from plants including olive and canola (rapeseed) oil. The polyunsaturated fats are also found in foods processed from plants including safflower, sunflower, corn, and soybean oils. When you substitute both the monounsaturated and polyunsaturated fats for saturated fats in your diet, you will help reduce your blood cholesterol.

How much cholesterol should I eat in one day?

Although the average American diet contains 350-450mg of cholesterol, it is best not to eat more than 300mg of cholesterol per day. Make sure that less than 30% of your calorie intake comes from fat. The average is 35% to 40%. If your cholesterol is in the high-risk range, reducing your total fat intake to 20-25% of your caloric intake will be helpful. If your cholesterol is high, you should increase the amount of protein and carbohydrates in your diet while you decrease your fat and cholesterol.

Where can I find more information about cholesterol and diets?

Your physician or clinic may be helpful. With the recent interest in cholesterol reducing diets, many publications are now available. In addition, the National Cholesterol Education Program (NCEP) recently published several excellent booklets entitled *So You Have High Blood Cholesterol, Eating To Lower Your High Blood Cholesterol* and *Community Guide to Cholesterol Resources*. These can be obtained free of charge by writing to:

National Cholesterol Education Program
National Heart, Lung, and Blood Institute
National Institutes of Health
C-200
Bethesda, MD 20892

Your local hospital is another source of information. If you cannot find a dietician in your community, call the Division of Practice of the American Dietetic Association at (312) 899-0040 for further information.

MENOPAUSE AND CARDIOVASCULAR DISEASE

How is menopause a risk factor for the development of atherosclerosis?

Scientific evidence shows that once you enter menopause, your chances of heart attack increase if your body lacks estrogen. This deficiency has been implicated as a high risk factor in the formation of atherosclerosis and coronary artery disease.

If I have an early menopause, will I have a higher risk of sustaining a heart attack?

Several studies performed since 1968 have shown that if you have an early menopause, either naturally occurring or surgically induced, your risk of heart attack appears to be at least three times as great as a woman of similar age who has not yet gone through menopause.

What causes the rise in coronary artery disease after menopause?

No one knows the exact mechanism, but it appears that one of the most important factors is an increase in cholesterol that occurs at that time. In addition, the lack of estrogen may have a direct effect on the integrity of the blood vessels, predisposing them to cholesterol deposits and plaque formation.

How does menopause affect lipid metabolism?

After menopause, your total cholesterol and low density lipoprotein (LDL) cholesterol increase. The triglyceride level also rises. These changes are felt to significantly increase the incidence of heart attacks at this time.

ESTROGEN REPLACEMENT AND CARDIOVASCULAR DISEASE

Can estrogen change my cholesterol and lower my chance for coronary artery disease?

Estrogen will influence the different types of cholesterol in your blood. As a rule, the estrogens used in postmenopausal estrogen replacement therapy (*conjugated equine estrogen, estradiol,* and *estrone*) cause a decrease in LDL-cholesterol and a rise in HDL-cholesterol, both very positive factors in preventing coronary artery disease. Several studies have shown that women who take the recommended doses of estrogen after their menopause not only have a lower heart attack rate, but also have a lower mortality rate from heart attacks.

I was told in the past that taking estrogen may increase my chance of cardiovascular disease. Is this true?

The *Framingham Study,* published approximately 25 years ago, did show a small rise in the incidence of cardiovascular disease in postmenopausal women who were on estrogen. The number of women that fell into the postmenopausal heart attack category was very small, however, and that part of the study was later found to be invalid. A number of new studies published in recent years (the *Nurses' Health Study* and the *Lipid Research Clinics Follow-Up Study*) have monitored large numbers of women. These investigations have shown a marked decrease (50–70%) of fatal cardiovascular disease in estrogen users.

Unfortunately, studies showing an increase in cardiovascular disease in women who took the birth control pill add to the confusion.

If the birth control pill increases my chance of a heart attack, why doesn't estrogen replacement therapy?

There are two explanations: The synthetic estrogen used in oral contraceptives, *ethinyl estradiol,* is about one hundred times more potent than the natural estrogens used in estrogen replacement therapy. Unlike the birth control pill, the natural estrogens in postmenopausal therapy cause a *decrease* in cardiovascular disease, not an increase. The second explanation involves the other major hormone in the pill, the progestational agent. Some progestational agents counteract the beneficial effects of estrogen by raising the LDL cholesterol in the blood, thereby causing an increase in atherosclerosis and cardiovascular disease. In fact, much of the negative impact of oral contraceptives is due to the progestational agent in the pill and not to the estrogen at all. Most of this data comes from studies that used the older, high-dose birth control pills. The present low-dose birth control pills do not have this negative influence.

How do the progestational agents affect the blood cholesterol?

Most of them have an effect on cholesterol that is opposite to that of estrogen: they cause a rise in the LDL-cholesterol and a fall in the HDL-cholesterol. Thus the addition of a progestational agent to the estrogen may counteract some of the potential benefits in terms of cardiovascular risk. One must evaluate the combination of the two hormones before concluding what their total effect will be on the cholesterol. Studies on the combination of estrogen and progestin in the present low-dose regimens do not show a deleterious effect on the lipid profile.

Do all the available progestational agents have the same effect?

The effect of progestational agents on cholesterol is related to the dosage. The lowest dose of progesterone that will counteract estrogen's effect on the uterine lining should be used. Medroxyprogesterone acetate (Provera, Amen, Cycrin, Curretabs), the most commonly used medication, used to be prescribed in a 10mg daily dose, but 5mg and possibly 2.5mg have been shown to counteract the negative effects of estrogen on the uterine lining.

In addition, a progesterone not yet available in the United States, micronized progesterone, has been shown (in a 200mg dose), to have no significant effect on blood cholesterol. Two new progestational agents, norgestimate and gestodene, have recently been released in birth control pills and also have been shown to have little effect on cholesterol. Once people have more experience with them, they most likely will be used in low-dose hormonal replacement therapy.

Why should I take progesterone if it may increase my risk of cardiovascular disease?

The progestational agent protects the uterine lining from the continuous stimulation of estrogen so *endometrial hyperplasia* and endometrial cancer (cancer of the uterine lining) will not develop from estrogen therapy. It may also help prevent the development of breast cancer, but this is very controversial among researchers. On the other hand, progesterone may counteract part of the beneficial effects estrogen alone has on lipid metabolism. Recent studies show that the combination of estrogen and progesterone in the low doses presently used does have beneficial effects.

The present recommendations are as follows: If you have your uterus, you should take progesterone along with the estrogen, but in as low a dose as possible. If you have had a hysterectomy (removal of the uterus), you do not need the progesterone (as the benefit of preventing breast cancer is not established) because it may have a negative effect on your blood cholesterol. Your cholesterol should be monitored while you are on estrogen-progesterone therapy, and if there is any significant change, an adjustment in the dosage should be considered.

Are the other risk factors for coronary artery disease affected by menopause?

Menopause impacts other risk factors for coronary artery disease to differing degrees. Menopause and estrogen replacement therapy may influence clotting tendency, sugar metabolism, blood pressure, and may increase the negative effects of cigarette smoking.

How does menopause affect the clotting of blood?

Estrogen has a tendency to increase the clotting capabilities of the blood. When you go through menopause, your blood becomes less able to form clots. A woman on estrogen replacement therapy will have a slight increase in her blood coagulability, but no greater than will a premenopausal woman. In contrast, women on oral contraceptives have an increased tendency to form blood clots *(thrombophlebitis)*, although much less so if they are taking the present low-dose birth control pills that have replaced higher-dose pills.

What causes the increased incidence of blood clots in women who take oral contraceptives?

The estrogen in oral contraceptives is *ethinyl estradiol*, a much more potent estrogen than those recommended for post-menopausal women. Ethinyl estradiol stimulates the liver proteins to increase their production of several of the clotting factors. This causes an increase in the incidence of thrombophlebitis in women who are taking the birth control pill.

The natural estrogens used in postmenopausal therapy *do not affect* the clotting factors. Very low doses (5µg, or 5 micrograms) of ethinyl estradiol have effects on the clotting mechanism that are similar to those of the natural estrogens, and are being used in postmenopausal therapy.

How does estrogen affect sugar metabolism?

The estrogen in oral contraceptives had an adverse affect on sugar metabolism. Estrogen replacement therapy does not have the same effect. The difference again is in the type and amount of estrogen in the birth control pill and that recommended for postmenopausal therapy. The present lower-dose birth control pills have a much smaller effect on sugar metabolism than did the previously used higher-dose pills.

I've heard the birth control pill can cause high blood pressure (hypertension). Is this also true of estrogen replacement therapy?

For some women, the ethinyl estradiol in the pill increases the production of another liver protein, *renin substrate (angiotensinogen)*, causing hypertension. The increased production of angiotensinogen *does not* occur with the types and amounts of estrogen used in postmenopausal therapy. In fact, several studies have shown postmenopausal women on estrogen therapy have lower blood pressures compared to women not on estrogen therapy.

Can I take estrogen if I have high blood pressure?

There is a tendency for your blood pressure to rise as you get older. Estrogen may actually be beneficial to you if you have hypertension. Reports have shown a lowering of blood pressure after estrogen replacement therapy is started. Your blood pressure should be monitored closely, however, to make sure you don't react adversely to medications. The patch may be a better form of estrogen for someone with high blood pressure, to avoid the first pass of estrogen through the liver (see pages 226–227).

Does smoking during menopause increase my predisposition to coronary artery disease?

Yes. Smoking is a risk factor for the development of coronary artery disease. If you smoke, you can expect to go through menopause several years earlier than if you do not smoke. Since an earlier menopause is also a risk factor for coronary artery disease, smoking is a double risk. If you smoke, you also are at higher risk of developing osteoporosis (See Chapter 8).

If the types of estrogen used in menopausal women have so few side effects, why are they not used in the birth control pill?

The amount of estrogen used in postmenopausal therapy is insufficient to suppress ovulation, so this dosage cannot be used in the birth control pill. Estrogen in oral contraceptives has been decreasing over the years, but it still requires 20–35μg (micrograms) of ethinyl estradiol to prevent ovulation. This lower dose has reduced the side effects of the pill quite markedly over the last few years, but it is still much more than the postmenopausal woman needs. The dose of ethinyl estradiol equivalent to 0.625mg of Premarin or 1mg of Estrace is approximately 5μg (micrograms). Therefore the 30–35μg of ethinyl estradiol in most low-dose birth control pills is still six to seven times more potent than the standard dose of postmenopausal hormones.

10

Can I Prevent
Wrinkled Skin?

The skin is one of the largest organs in our bodies and is very sensitive to changes that occur during the menopausal years. Many changes are inevitable while others can be delayed or prevented with appropriate hormonal therapy. During menopause, the small blood vessels under the very superficial layer of skin (the *epidermis*) are responsible for the menopausal hot flash. Skin thickness also starts decreasing with age and becomes more pronounced. Dry, flaky, easily stretched, wrinkled skin that bruised more readily used to be attributed to the normal aging process. Recent research indicates, however, that you can prevent much of this "normal" aging by maintaining an adequate hormonal level.

THE SKIN

What is skin?

The skin is considered an organ, just like other organs in your body, such as the lungs, liver, and heart. It is made up of a thin, outer layer called the *epidermis* and a deeper part called the *dermis*. The epidermis contains both *keratinocytes* (the *keratin* producing cells) and pigment-producing cells called *melanocytes* that become stimulated to create a tan upon exposure to the sun. Keratin produced by the epidermis gives a protective covering for the dermis.

What is the function of the dermis?

The dermis makes up the bulk of the skin and contains its vital structures. Ninety-seven percent of the dermis is composed of the protein, *collagen*. The remainder is made up of elastin fibers. Blood vessels, hair follicles, sweat and oil (*sebaceous*) glands, lymph vessels, sensory corpuscles, and autonomic and sensory nerves can all be found within the dermis.

What is collagen?

Collagen is a fibrous protein. The skin, bone, tendons, ligaments, *fascia* (a thick covering over our abdominal muscles), arteries, and the uterus contain about 90% of the body's supply. Collagen makes up the majority of the dermis. It is responsible for the elasticity, thickness, and tone of the skin.

HOW THE SKIN AGES

What happens to the collagen in my skin as I get older?

Collagen is constantly being destroyed and replaced. As you become older, more collagen tends to be destroyed than manufactured, so the skin becomes thinner and begins to fold on itself causing wrinkles. The collagen also loses some of its moisture, causing the skin to be drier. The collagen content decreases in postmenopausal women at an approximate rate of 2% per year. The muscle and fat tissue beneath the skin also

Figure 10-1

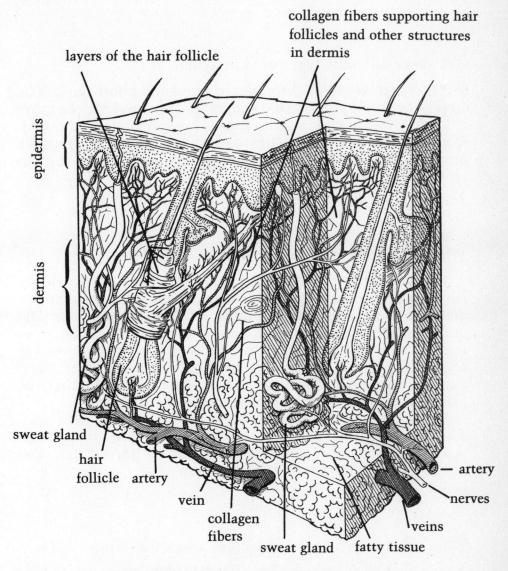

layers of the hair follicle

collagen fibers supporting hair
follicles and other structures
in dermis

epidermis

dermis

sweat gland

hair
follicle   artery

vein

collagen
fibers

sweat gland

artery

nerves

veins

fatty tissue

Cross section of skin showing complex makeup
with many stuctures.

tend to contract and shrink with age, resulting in skin that is stretched and folded upon itself (wrinkles).

Are there different types of skin aging?

Yes, there are two: chronologic aging and photoaging. The first is a normal process that occurs with age and may be more related to estrogen status than was previously thought. Photoaging is due to exposure to ultraviolet light rays from the sun. These processes intermingle and account for the changes in your skin as you grow older.

What effect does the sun have on the skin?

The sun removes needed moisture from the skin, accelerating the aging process by several years. Overexposure to the sun destroys the oil producing glands, as well as the elastin and collegen fibers. The latter appear to be especially sensitive to the sun's rays and account for the loss of elasticity, as well as the yellow discoloration seen in those who have been overexposed to the sun for a number of years. Marked wrinkling also becomes prominent as a result of photoaging.

Sun exposure also predisposes you to several skin conditions that can be precancerous (*actinic keratosis*), or it can act as an outright cause of skin cancer (*basal cell* and *squamous cell carcinomas* of the skin).

What other environmental factors affect the skin?

Smoking is detrimental to the skin. Nicotine causes premature aging by constricting the blood vessels. This decreases needed oxygen. Rapid weight loss and living in a dry environment are also deleterious to young looking skin.

What is the effect of estrogen on the skin?

Estrogen plays an important role in skin metabolism. It is responsible for fat distribution within the dermis, giving the skin its support and firmness. It helps retain water in the skin. This explains why fluid retention occurs if one takes excessive estrogen. This hormone also helps maintain the thickness of skin through its effect on collagen, the major protein in skin.

How does estrogen affect collagen?

Estrogen is necessary for the production of collagen. Studies comparing skin collagen and skin thickness have been performed in postmenopausal women on estrogen therapy and those not on estrogen therapy. These have consistently shown that women on estrogen had thicker skin with a higher collagen content; they had fewer wrinkles and moister skin.

WHAT FACTORS AFFECT HOW MY SKIN WILL AGE?

If I take estrogen after I've already developed wrinkles, will it help them go away?

Not only can the aging process be stopped, but some collagen can be replaced and the wrinkles reduced with estrogen replacement. The improvement will be self-limiting however, as there appears to be a maximum amount of collagen that can be produced in each individual. A certain degree of collagen loss occurs with age regardless of the estrogen content of the skin.

Does the age at which I undergo menopause determine how my skin will look?

Women who go through a later menopause will have younger looking, less wrinkled skin (because they have been producing estrogen for a longer period of time) than women who go through an early menopause.

Do women who are heavier usually have younger looking skin?

In general, if you are heavy, your skin will look younger than a thin woman's. And, conversely, if you are very thin, your skin will wrinkle at an earlier age than someone who is overweight. Women who have more fat produce more estrogen because their body fat converts some of the androgenic hormones from the adrenal gland and ovaries to estrogen. (See Chapter 2.) The added estrogen protects against the development of wrinkles. In addition, women who have extra fat on their bodies will have an extra "fat pad," giving the skin more support.

Does heredity affect how my skin ages?

Heredity is important in most areas in medicine. A family history of young looking skin will be a benefit to you.

If I already have wrinkles and am postmenopausal, how long will it be before I notice a change in my skin if I start estrogen therapy?

Studies have shown that it takes about six months of physiological hormonal therapy to reconstitute skin collagen once it is lost.

Is skin collagen more closely correlated with my chronological age or the number of years I am past my menopause?

There is no apparent correlation between your *actual* age and the thickness or collagen content of your skin. There is a strong correlation between skin thickness and the collagen content of your skin, when it is compared to the number of years since menopause.

KEEPING YOUR SKIN YOUNGER LOOKING

Do collagen creams help restore collagen to the skin?

The expensive collagen creams have not been shown to improve the collagen content of the skin. Although many women swear by them and assert that their skin has fewer wrinkles, this effect is probably related to the other moisturizing qualities of the creams and not from the collagen they contain. The same effect could be achieved from a much less expensive product.

What can I do to keep my skin young and wrinkle free?

Maintaining a youthful appearance is important to all of us. No one likes to show her age, and having young looking, wrinkle-free skin is important in maintaining that youthful appearance. The following has been shown to be helpful in achieving that goal.

- **Avoid the sun and excessive tanning as much as possible. It may look nice in the short term, but over many years, excessive sun exposure will increase your potential for developing wrinkles.**

- **If you are overweight and plan to reduce, do so slowly. Rapid weight loss will cause your skin to lose much of its support. This can actually increase the chance of wrinkles. With a slow, steady weight loss, your skin is able to adjust. It contracts gradually without the wrinkling effect.**

- Keep your skin moist! This is one of the most important factors. Maintaining adequate humidity in your home and work environment is important especially if you live in a dry climate. The winter season in northern climates can also be very dry and the use of humidifiers in your home will help. Moisturizers prevent water loss from the skin. Many soaps are drying and should be avoided in favor of cleansing creams, especially for the face and neck.

- Sufficient fluid intake is important. You should drink between six and eight glasses of water a day to maintain adequate hydration for the collagen in the dermis of the skin.

- Exercise regularly—it improves circulation to the skin as well as tones your muscles for general well being.

- An adequate diet that includes protein, minerals and vitamins, especially Vitamin C, has been shown to be important in collagen synthesis.

- If you smoke, stop.

- If you are lacking estrogen and have other reasons to be on estrogen replacement, hormone therapy will be beneficial in preventing further wrinkles as well as restoring some of the collagen that has already been lost.

Should I take estrogen just to prevent wrinkles?

Estrogen is a medication that has potential benefits and side effects. It should not be taken solely to prevent wrinkles, but there may be an association between wrinkles and other estrogen-deprivation syndromes, such as osteoporosis and a higher incidence of cardiovascular disease. If this proves to be true, and if other postmenopasual symptoms are present, estrogen may be of benefit.

What is Retin-A and can it prevent wrinkles?

Retin-A is the brand name for *tretinoin*. It is a drug that has been available in the U.S. for the treatment of *acne vulgaris*, a deforming acne condition of the face. A recent study published in the *Journal of the American Medical Association* showed that tretinoin can reverse photoaging that has already developed. It is a cream that is applied in small quantities on the area to be treated. A marked inflammation and redness (*dermatitis*) develops which caused several people in the study to stop using the drug. The study showed that the tretinoin-treated faces decreased fine wrinkles and, to a lesser extent, coarse wrinkles, resulting in a healthier glow to the treated skin. If you are considering *Retin-A*, you should only use it under the directions of a physician or dermatologist (skin doctor) who has experience with its use.

Can anything else be done to reduce the number of wrinkles I have?

Surgery, such as face lift operations, *suction lipectomies* and *dermabrasions*, performed by plastic surgeons or dermatologists who specialize in cosmetic surgery can reduce the number of wrinkles. These are not permanent cures and may have to be repeated if the wrinkles continue to upset you as the aging process progresses.

THE CONNECTION BETWEEN SKIN AND BONES

Is there a correlation between the condition of my skin and the chance of my developing osteoporosis?

Studies have suggested that if you have good-looking skin with good collagen and thickness, your bones will be in the same shape and less likely to develop osteoporosis. Collagen is present in both tissues. If there is a loss of collagen in one organ, there may be a parallel loss in the other.

Why is the correlation between the condition of the skin and bone collagen important?

It may be a fairly simple way of predicting which women will be more susceptible to osteoporotic bone fractures. Further studies are necessary in this area to confirm this initial impression.

PERSPIRATION, UNWANTED HAIR LOSS AND HAIR GROWTH

Why do I perspire more since I finished menstruating?

Androgens (the male hormones all women have) stimulate the sweat glands located within the dermis of the skin. During the menstrual years, when estrogen was being produced, it counteracted the effect of the androgens on the sweat glands, controlling the amount of sweat they produced. After menopause, the androgens are unopposed by estrogen resulting in an increase in perspiration. Estrogen replacement therapy should prevent the increased sweating during the postmenopausal period.

Does menopause cause hair loss?

Some women do notice a thinning of their hair after menopause. The hair follicle (the place where each individual hair has its root) is located deep within the dermis. The tissue surrounding the hair follicles is mostly made up of collagen which gives it support. Menopause does result in less support to the hair follicle, increasing the tendency for hair loss. (See illustration of the skin on page 162.)

Will estrogen replacement therapy prevent hair loss?

Estrogen replacement therapy will counteract most of the affects of menopause on the hair follicle.

Does estrogen affect hair in other ways?

Estrogen affects the hair on the body in different ways. Hair located on the face, pubic area and under the arms are referred to as *sexual hair*. Estrogen stimulates the growth of sexual hair and inhibits hair growth on other parts of the body, such as the chest, arms, and legs. During the menopausal years, some women may note hair loss in the sexual areas as well as an increase in hair in other places. A lack of estrogen also causes the hair, themselves, to become coarser and dryer. Estrogen may be of benefit in preventing hair loss which occurs with normal aging because of its support to the hair follicle.

Why do some women grow a beard after menopause?

As ovarian estrogen production decreases and eventually stops, the androgens produced by the adrenal glands and ovaries are unopposed by estrogen. As a result, there may be an increase in male hair distribution in some areas of the body such as on the face, arms, and legs. This is not as bad as it sounds. Usually only a few coarse hairs may grow on the chin or side of the face (not an entire beard) five to ten years after menopause.

If I take estrogen, will it prevent unwanted hair growth?

Estrogen counteracts the effect of androgens on the hair follicles. It may take several months before you notice the beneficial effect.

11

Will I Get Breast Cancer?

Fibrocystic breast disease and breast cancer are prevalent in the perimenopausal and postmenopausal female. You may be confused if you have been told that you have fibrocystic breasts or that your breast feels a "little cystic." What does this mean? Are you going to get breast cancer? In this chapter, I will clarify your questions about this condition.

Breast cancer is the most common female cancer. It afflicts one out of nine women. Because of its frequency, you most likely know someone who has this disease or you may have lost a friend or relative to it. Breast cancer causes some confusion. There is conflicting evidence as to who is at high risk and what role diet and hormones play. I will explain breast cancer, its risk factors, and the relationship between this disease and hormonal replacement therapy.

THE BREAST

What does breast tissue consist of?

The breast is the mammary gland common to all mammals. It consists of a *glandular* and *ductal* system surrounded by varying amounts of fat, connective tissue, blood vessels, nerves and lymphatics called *stroma*. A number of glands merge to form *lobules* which converge into a system of ducts that drain out at the nipple.

Does the breast respond to the hormones involved in the menstrual cycle?

Yes. The breast is very responsive to the estrogen and progesterone produced by the ovaries during the normal menstrual cycle. At puberty, these hormones stimulate the breast to develop and grow. During the first two weeks of the menstrual cycle, estrogen induces minimal activity within the glandular system of the breast, but after ovulation, with the addition of progesterone, the combined hormones cause a marked swelling of the cells and fluid within the breast. This is why some women experience premenstrual breast tenderness. It indicates that they are producing progesterone and are ovulating with their menstrual cycles. Women with fibrocystic breast disease may experience premenstrual breast tenderness as well, but the pain and tenderness may be more severe and last longer than normal premenstrual breast discomfort.

What happens to the breast during pregnancy?

During pregnancy, with its associated increase in both estrogen and progesterone, the glandular, as well as the stromal, components of the breast tissue enlarge, often quite markedly. After delivery, the cells of the glandular system begin producing milk.

What happens to the breast after pregnancy and lactation (nursing)?

After lactation, the breast suffers a loss of elasticity and tends to become prolapsed as milk no longer is produced. The glandular portion and the major ducts are much more easily felt because of the loss of surrounding fat. As a result, some areas of the breast may feel like a cord or a small piece of rope.

FIBROCYSTIC BREAST DISEASE

What is fibrocystic breast disease?

Fibrocystic breast disease is really not a "disease" per se but a catchall phrase used to describe one of approximately 50 different benign breast conditions. The actual medical names of these conditions are unimportant for our purposes. Any time a breast examination is performed and the breasts feel "lumpy," the breast is referred to as being cystic and a diagnosis of fibrocystic breast disease is made. Some of the different diagnoses are actually variations of normal breast tissue, while others are pathologic and deserve closer attention. True cystic breast disease is present when a cyst becomes prominent and fills with fluid.

How common is fibrocystic breast disease?

As many as 40% to 60% of all women's breasts feel "cystic" and meet the criteria for a diagnosis of fibrocystic breast disease. Indeed, it is truly impossible to accurately evaluate the incidence of this disease since its definition is so broad. When the breast is examined under the microscope, either by biopsy specimen or studies performed at autopsy, as many as 90% of all women have breast tissue that meets the pathologic diagnosis of fibrocystic breast disease.

What are the symptoms of fibrocystic breast disease?

Pain, nodularity and tenderness in the breasts are the classic symptoms. Most occur premstrually only, but in more severe cases, the symptoms can last all month long. Occasionally, a well-defined cyst filled with a clear or murky-green fluid may form.

If I have fibrocystic breast disease will I have a greater chance of getting breast cancer?

Because the diagnosis of fibrocystic breast disease is so common and so vague, it is difficult to evaluate different studies that have been performed on the relationship between breast cancer and cystic disease of the breast. Some studies have shown no correlation with cancer, while others show a two- to fivefold increased risk for breast cancer.

How is fibrocystic breast disease treated?

The treatments fall into five categories: diet, hormonal manipulation, diuretic and pain medication, and surgery.

DIET AND FIBROCYSTIC BREAST DISEASE

Which dietary measures can help fibrocystic breast disease?

Decreasing caffeine and dietary fat while increasing Vitamin E and the Vitamin B complex has helped some woemn.

Do all physicians believe that the dietary factors help?

The dietary measures may or may not be helpful to all women. The medical literature is equivocal. Some researchers show diet makes a difference, while others have attributed benefits to a placebo effect. Caffeine is the most common dietary factor associated with fibrocystic breast disease.

What are the most common foods that contain caffeine?

Coffee, tea, chocolate, cocoa and colas are the greatest sources of caffeine in your diet. You may notice a marked improvement in your breast tenderness and pain when you decrease your caffeine intake gradually over a period of time. If you want to give this treatment the best chance of working, you should completely eliminate caffeine from your diet.

Figure 11-1

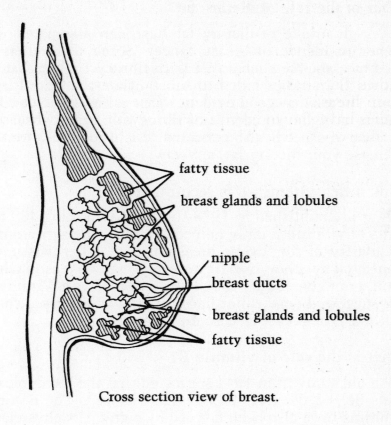

fatty tissue

breast glands and lobules

nipple

breast ducts

breast glands and lobules

fatty tissue

Cross section view of breast.

Should I stop my caffeine intake suddenly?

It is best to do so gradually rather than abruptly. If you are consuming a significant amount of caffeine (the equivalent of six to twelve cups of coffee a day) and stop suddenly, you will probably get severe caffeine withdrawal headaches similar to migraines. It is best to ease off caffeine over a period of several weeks. In fact, if you ever fast for a 24 hour period (as on some religious holidays) the headache you develop is usually from caffeine withdrawal and is unrelated to hunger.

What is the role of dietary fat?

A high intake of dietary fat has been associated with a higher incidence of breast cancer. Some researchers have tired to associate such a diet with fibrocystic breast disease, but further studies failed to substantiate the initial impression. There is no good evidence that a high-fat diet contributes to a higher incidence of fibrocystic breast disease, but because of other health concerns, it is a good idea for you to decrease your dietary fat, anyway.

How much vitamin E is recommended?

A study published in 1978 showed that taking 400 to 800 units of vitamin E daily helped diminish the symptoms and nodularity of fibrocystic breast disease. This was not substantiated by other investigators, but I see no reason why you should not give it a try to see if it will help you. Vitamin E in the suggested dose is not harmful, and it has eased the pain of fibrocystic breast disease for many women.

What is the role of vitamin B?

An old study from 1944 suggested that the B complex vitamins helped the liver metabolize estrogen. The B complex vitamins have also been favored by a group of physicians for the treatment of Premenstrual Syndrome and for this reason may be helpful in decreasing the tenderness associated with fibrocystic breast disease. All of these dietary measures may not be helpful to all women, but they seem rather harmless to try before going to other measures. Vitamin B_6 (pyridoxine) appears to be the most helpful, in a dose of 100mg per day.

OTHER TREATMENTS FOR FIBROCYSTIC BREAST DISEASE

Can medications help the swelling and tenderness of my breasts

A diuretic taken a week to ten days before the onset of your menstrual period may relieve the breast tenderness. An anti-inflammatory and anti-prostaglandin drug such as ibuprofen (Advil, Nuprin, Medipren, Motrin) in a dose of 400mg three times a day may also help.

What are the hormonal measures to control fibrocystic breast disease?

The use of oral contraceptives, androgens, an anti-estrogen medication called *tamoxifen* (a drug used to treat women with positive estrogen receptor breast cancer), and *danazol* (the medication used to treat endometriosis) have all been used to treat fibrocystic breast disease. Each of these medications works, but they have their own side effects, such as hot flashes, weight gain, nausea, fluid retention, and *amenorrhea* (no menstrual periods). Consult your physician if you feel your symptoms warrant the use of any of these medications.

What is the surgical treatment of fibrocystic breast disease?

If a well-defined cyst is present, your physician will aspirate it with a needle to collapse the cyst and examine the fluid. Most of the time, cystic breast fluid is light or murky green. It can be sent to the laboratory for analysis, but not all physicians find this helpful.

Aspirating the cyst will usually relieve the pain immediately and will also relieve your fear that the cyst was a cancerous tumor. If the cyst fluid is bloody, or if a well-defined lump is still present after the aspiration, a biopsy of the lump should be performed. Fibrocystic breast disease lumps are usually painful and tender. Cancerous lumps are often asymptomatic.

What are other indications for a breast biopsy?

A sudden increase in a lump that is being followed, any persistent redness or dimpling of the skin, a bloody discharge from the nipple, or a lump that concerns you or your physician are all indications for a breast biopsy.

BREAST CANCER

What is cancer?

Cancer is an abnormal growth of cells which results in formation of a lump or tumor. If these cancer cells spread to another part of the body, they continue to multiply, destroying and replacing normal tissue. If the organ destroyed is vital to life, such as the lung, brain, or liver, death will eventually ensue.

Which cells in the breast cause cancer?

Any of the cells may become cancerous, but the most common form of breast cancer involves the cells of the gland lobules and ductal system. The majority of breast cancer originates within the ductal system. Other, less common forms of breast cancer may start from the cells in the skin around the nipple, the sebaceous glands around the hair follicles, the sweat glands, or any other cells within the stroma of the breast.

How does breast cancer spread?

Breast cancer spreads by direct extension, in the bloodstream, and most commonly, by way of the lymphatic system. If breast cancer spreads by direct extension, it may cause an ulceration of the skin over the breast, or it may grow into and through the muscle overlying the ribs and attach to the rib cage. If breast cancer erodes into a small artery or vein, it can spread in the blood stream to any organ in the body. Most often, the cancer goes into the lymph nodes under the arm and then into the general lymphatic system, and eventually into the bloodstream and general circulation.

Which organs are most affected by the spread of breast cancer?

Breast cancer may spread to anywhere in the body, but the major sites of *metastasis* (the spread of disease from one site to another) are the bones (spine, long bones, skull, and pelvis), lung, brain, and liver.

How common is breast cancer?

Breast cancer will occur in about 10% of all women.

How many women die from breast cancer each year?

In 1992, the American Cancer Society estimated that breast cancer started in 180,000 new patients and caused 46,000 deaths. One in 30 women will die of this disease. It is presently the second leading cause of cancer deaths in women in the U.S., with cancer of the lung just recently surpassing breast cancer and the leading cause. (This is related to the increase in smoking by women during the last 20 to 30 years.) It is unfortunate, but despite all the recent advances in mammography and cancer treatment, the mortality rate of breast cancer has not changed during the past 50 years. Early detection remains the main hope of decreasing the mortality rate of breast cancer.

RISK FACTORS FOR BREAST CANCER

Are certain women more prone to breast cancer than others?

Women who live in Denmark, England, Scotland, Israel, Netherlands, Switzerland, and Canada have slightly higher breast cancer rates than women in the U.S. Women from Asia, especially Japan, have a much lower incidence of breast cancer. As women from Asia migrate to Hawaii and the United

States, however, their risk for breast cancer increases, indicating that an environmental or dietary factor contributes to the higher risk in the United States.

What are the risk factors for breast cancer?

Although we can talk about various risk factors associated with breast cancer, I must emphasize that in approximately 80% of all breast cancers, there is no identifiable factor which we normally attribute to cancer risk. The known risk factors have been divided into several categories: dietary, radiation, hereditary, and hormonal.

DIET AND BREAST CANCER RISK

Do certain foods contribute to a higher risk for breast cancer?

Over the years, several dietary factors including caffeine, dietary fat, vitamins A and E, and alcohol have all been tied to breast cancer risk.

Is caffeine associated with a higher risk for breast cancer?

In 1980, a study showed a possible link between the *methylxanthines* (substances common to any food containing caffeine), and fibrocystic breast disease and possibly cancer. Several years later, subsequent investigations did not support the findings of the earlier study, especially in relation to cancer. Although many women who eliminate caffeine containing foods such as chocolate, coffee, tea, and colas from their diet do seem to have fewer symptoms of fibrocystic breast disease, they do not appear, at least at present, to enjoy a lower incidence of breast cancer.

Does dietary fat contribute to a higher risk for breast cancer?

The association of a high fat diet with a greater risk for breast cancer originates chiefly from animal studies. When different population groups are studied for breast cancer risk, however, women who eat low fat diets (Asian women) do appear to have a lower incidence of breast cancer. Also, various religious groups that are practicing vegetarians enjoy a lower incidence of breast cancer. A large study of almost a 100,000 women, however, failed to show a relationship between cholesterol levels and breast cancer, so if there is an increased risk associated with a high fat diet, it is not correlated with the cholesterol level.

The National Cancer Institute has proposed a national multicenter study to settle this issue. The Institute wants to have a group of women who are at high risk for breast cancer reduce the calories they obtain from dietary fat from 40% (the average U.S. norm) to 20%. The study will then monitor these women for the next 10 years to determine if diet makes a difference.

Reducing the total fat in your diet is beneficial, as it decreases your risk for coronary artery disease. Even if it turns out that fat is not associated with breast cancer, it is a good idea to reduce the total fat in your diet for other health reasons.

Is a vitamin deficiency associated with a greater risk of breast cancer?

A lack of both vitamins A and E has been implicated in a higher risk of breast cancer. One study showed a fivefold increase in risk associated with a low blood level of vitamin E. Further studies are needed to substantiate this association.

Is alcohol consumption associate with an increased risk for breast cancer?

A study from 1987 showed that women who consume even a modest amount of alcohol (a daily glass of wine) may risk a higher incidence of breast cancer. It is not certain whether additional studies will substantiate this association. It may be best to decrease your alcohol intake if breast cancer is a concern for you.

What can be concluded about the dietary factors implicated with breast cancer?

Although a correlation between dietary factors and breast cancer is suggested, the nature and significance of the association is not yet established and awaits further studies. The suggested dietary factors are good general health measures to follow even if it turns out there is no link with breast cancer.

RADIATION AND BREAST CANCER RISK

Is radiation exposure a risk factor for breast cancer?

Exposure to ionizing radiation increases the risk of developing breast cancer in women. Studies from atomic bomb survivors in Japan showed a higher incidence of breast cancer in women who were exposed to a high dose of radiation. Years ago, women were treated with radiation for postpartum mastitis (a breast infection following childbirth) and tuberculosis. Each of these groups of women were found to have a higher incidence of breast cancer as they were followed over the next 20 years. Women who were employed as radium dial workers before 1930 also were found to have a 50% greater risk of dying from breast cancer compared to the general population.

Does the age at time of the radiation exposure make a difference?

Exposure during adolescence is associated with a greater risk than exposure at later ages.

If I have routine mammograms according to the recommendations of the American Cancer Society, will I increase my chance of developing breast cancer?

Although mammography does expose you to some radiation, it is minuscule compared to the doses emitted in the above mentioned studies. The X-ray should be performed by the new, low dose mammography machines that have been developed in the last few years. The benefit from a mammography exam far outweighs the risk of exposure. The risk should not be of great concern to you.

HEREDITY AND BREAST CANCER RISK

Does heredity play a role in the development of breast cancer?

Heredity plays a definite role in breast cancer. In order for a cancer to be considered *hereditary*, a definite linkage through many generations must be established. If the linkage cannot be established, but the disease is in the family, then breast cancer is considered *familial* but not hereditary. About 5% of all breast cancers can be traced to a direct genetic linkage over many generations. An additional 13% are familial—they tend to run in a family, but not strongly enough to meet the hereditary criteria. In other words, about 18% of all breast cancers will have a family history, while 82% will be sporadic, without a familial history. The 5% estimate of hereditary breast cancer may be conservative, however, because as time goes by, some of the sporadic and familial cases may become part of the hereditary pattern.

What are the clinical features of hereditary breast cancer?

The features of a true hereditary breast cancer are described below.

- **Hereditary breast cancer occurs earlier with the average age being 44, compared to about 60 for sporadic cases.**

- There is a higher incidence of bilateral (both breasts) cancer in hereditary breast cancer, with as many as 46% of the patients eventually having cancer in both breasts.

- There is a higher incidence of other associated cancers, such as ovary, brain, lung, colon, adrenal gland, thyroid, and leukemia with hereditary breast cancer.

- Hereditary breast cancer tends to be passed on as an autosomal dominant mode of inheritance. This means that your father's family history is as important as your mother's. A male may pass the gene on to his daughter. It is therefore important to inquire about *both* maternal and paternal family histories as far back as possible to determine if the hereditary type of breast cancer is present.

It appears that hereditary breast cancer may be passed on by a specific gene. With improvements in genetic research, it may be possible to identify those young women who are at high risk for breast cancer prior to any clinical symptoms.

Do men get breast cancer?

Men can get breast cancer, but it is 100 times more common in women than in men.

How do I know if I am at high risk for breast cancer?

If you have a first-degree relative (parents, siblings, and children) with the hereditary features of breast cancer, you are considered at the highest risk. If you have second-degree relatives (both maternal and paternal grandparents, aunts, and uncles) with the hereditary features of breast cancer, you also would be considered a risk, but not as high. If you have both first and second degree relatives with an early age onset of breast cancer, you may be at a 50% risk of eventually developing this disease.

If I have a strong family history of breast cancer, should I be monitored more closely than other women?

Yes, you should. If you have a family history of breast cancer, you have about a 15-20% risk of cancer, and if both first and second-degree relatives developed breast cancer at an early age, you may be at a 50% risk. You should:

- **be instructed on how to perform self-breast examinations at an early age**
- **see your primary physician every six months rather than once a year for a careful breast exam**
- **have a baseline mammogram as early as age 25 and then every two or three years thereafter**

In some cases, where the family history is extremely strong with a mother, grandmother, and sister all developing early age breast cancer, consideration for a *prophylactic subcutaneous mastectomy* should be given.

What is a prophylactic subcutaneous mastectomy?

It is an operation in which the majority of the breast tissue is removed while the skin and nipple over the breast are preserved. Breast implants are placed beneath the skin of the breast. There are no adequate studies to demonstrate that a subcutaneous mastectomy reduces the incidence of breast cancer. This operation should only be performed after appropriate consultation with a genetic counselor and your husband and after you have obtained a second surgical opinion.

HORMONES AND BREAST CANCER RISK

What are the possible hormonal risk factors associated with breast cancer?

The following hormonal causes have been associated with a higher incidence of breast cancer:

- **early age at menarche**
- **late age at menopause**
- **increased postmenopausal weight**
- **nulliparity (never giving birth)**
- **late age at first full-term delivery**

Artificial menopause prior to your natural menopause is associated with a decreased risk of breast cancer.

Does age at menarche affect the risk for breast cancer?

Several studies have confirmed a higher risk of breast cancer for women with an early menarche (first menstrual period). If you had your first menstrual period at age 12 or younger, you have twice the risk of breast cancer as a woman who had her first menstrual period at age 13 or later. This effect is true for young women (age 32 and younger) and decreases with increasing age.

Does the regularity of my menstrual cycle determine a risk for breast cancer?

The earlier you established regular menstrual cycles, the greater the risk for breast cancer. A woman with early menarche (age 12 or less) and early establishment of regular menstrual cycles has a fourfold risk of breast cancer compared to a woman with a late menarche (age 13 or older) and a long duration of irregular cycles.

Does age at menopause affect risk for breast cancer?

If you experienced a natural menopause (your last menstrual period) at age 45, you have only one half the risk of suffering from breast cancer as a woman who entered menopause after age 55. Another way to look at this data: if you have 40 or more years of regular active menstruation you will have twice the risk of breast cancer as a woman who has had less than 30 years of active menstruation.

Does artificial menopause affect risk for breast cancer?

If your ovaries were removed surgically, or if they were destroyed by pelvic irradiation, you will have less risk of developing breast cancer than a woman of the same age going through a natural menopause.

Does weight affect the risk for breast cancer?

The risk of developing breast cancer increases 80% if you are over 60 years of age and approximately 20 pounds overweight. Increased weight in women younger than 50, however, does not appear to expose one to a greater risk. This mechanism is not fully understood, but it may be related to the body fat's production of estrogen after menopause.

Does the age at which I had my children affect my risk for breast cancer?

Earlier childbirth appears to exert a *protective* effect on the risk of breast cancer. If your first child was born when you were 19 or younger, you will have about half the risk of a woman who had her first child at 35 or older, or a woman who never had children at all.

Does the number of children I have affect my risk for breast cancer?

If you have never had children, you are at a greater risk for breast cancer than a woman with children. The more children you have, the less likely you are to get breast cancer. The difference in risk, however, does not appear to be great and may be related to when you gave birth to your first child rather than the number of children you have.

Does the amount of estrogen I produce affect the risk for breast cancer?

It is highly suggested that estrogen plays a role in the development of breast cancer. The more years you menstruate, the greater your risk for getting breast cancer. The exact mechanism of estrogen's role is not fully understood.

Do women with breast cancer have higher estrogen blood levels?

Several studies have shown that women with breast cancer do have higher estrogen blood levels when compared to women who do not have breast cancer. Obese women also have a higher incidence of breast cancer. Since the greatest source of estrogen after the menopause is the body fat, the increased incidence of breast cancer in obese women may be related to their higher estrogen levels.

What is prolactin?

Prolactin is a hormone produced by the pituitary gland that causes the breast to produce milk. Recent studies have shown that any drug which stimulates the production of prolactin causes an increase in breast tumors in mice and rats.

Are prolactin levels increased in women with breast cancer?

Studies have shown that premenopausal women who develop breast cancer do have higher levels of prolactin. In postmenopausal women, some studies have shown a significant elevation while others have shown no difference.

Does progesterone affect the risk of breast cancer?

The effect of progesterone on breast tissue is apparently different from its effect on the uterine lining. As discussed in

Chapter 2, progesterone counteracts the build-up of the uterine lining caused by estrogen. On the other hand, progesterone actually *stimulates* the breast cells to divide and tissue to develop. This process appears to reach its peak just prior to the menstrual period when progesterone is at its highest levels. Therefore, progesterone, at least in the presence of estrogen, appears to encourage cell proliferation and division in the breast. The presence of progesterone may explain why women with regular menstrual cycles have a higher incidence of breast cancer than those whose cycles are irregular. (Women with irregular cycles do not ovulate regularly and therefore, do not produce progesterone as often.)

Will my taking oral contraceptives (birth control pill), increase my risk for breast cancer?

Several studies have shown that there is no increased risk of breast cancer if you used birth control pills during most of your reproductive life. A few studies have indicated, however, that if oral contraceptives are used around the time of menopause (46 to 50 years of age), the risk of breast cancer may increase slightly.

These studies were performed with the higher-dose birth control pills in use years ago. The present commonly prescribed low-dose birth control pills are not associated with an increase in breast cancer if used by perimenopausal women.

What if I have fibrocystic breast disease or a family history of breast cancer and am on the birth control pill? Will that influence my risk for breast cancer?

Studies *do not* show a higher risk for breast cancer in this case. In fact, the pill may be of benefit to you, if you have severe symptoms of fibrocystic breast disease.

HORMONE REPLACEMENT AND BREAST CANCER

Does estrogen replacement therapy during the postmenopausal years increase breast cancer risk?

Several studies published around 1980 showed a slightly increased risk in breast cancer associated with estrogen use during the menopause. Other more recent studies have found no increase in risk in women who take estrogens or estrogen with progesterone during the menopause. The increase in risk reported earlier appears to be related to the higher doses of estrogen recommended during the 1970s and not to the present low dose regimens.

With conflicting data on published studies, what am I to believe?

Based on the best data available at the present, it appears that long-term use of estrogen replacement therapy in moderately high doses does carry with it a slight increase in breast cancer risk. Lower doses for a short period of time carry no measurable risk. The lower doses of estrogen for long periods of time have not been studied adequately to draw specific conclusions, but they appear not to carry much risk. Several recently published studies confirm the impression that the present recommended doses of estrogen during menopause do not increase the risk of postmenopausal breast cancer when all other risk factors are considered.

I've heard that progesterone may protect against the development of breast cancer. Is that true?

Some preliminary studies have shown that adding progesterone to estrogen in women who still have their uterus may actually increase protection against breast cancer and endometrial cancer. For this reason, some doctors are postulating that even if you do not have your uterus, you should take progesterone. It is still too early, however, to draw definitive conclusions from these studies. Most physicians still *do not* recommend progesterone unless you have your uterus because of the negative effect of the progestational agents on your lipids. This may increase your risk for coronary artery disease. (See Chapter 9 and 13.)

If I have regular checkups while I am taking estrogen, will I reduce my risk?

Data is beginning to come out indicating that women on estrogen or estrogen-progesterone therapy actually have a lower death rate from breast cancer than women not on hormonal replacement therapy. Women on estrogen therapy are usually monitored more closely by their physicians and have regular checkups and mammograms. This could be the reason for the difference in death rates. If breast cancer is found in an estrogen user, it is usually discovered at a much earlier stage, and thus the chance of catching and curing the cancer is greater. The protective effect of estrogen on the cardiovascular system may also account for better survival rates in women who are on estrogen therapy.

BREAST CANCER DETECTION WITH MAMMOGRAPHY

What can I do to detect breast cancer at the earliest possible stage?

There are three methods utilized to screen for early breast cancer: the breast self-examination (BSE), medical examination, and mammography. You should perform the breast self-examination monthly. Even if your breasts have a "cystic" feeling, you should get used to what they feel like so you can tell if there is a change. Your physician should perform a complete, careful, non-rushed breast examination during your yearly physical. A recent study did show that a good portion of breast lumps were missed by physicians during a rushed exam. Mammography should be performed on a regular basis.

What is a mammography?

Mammography is an X-ray procedure used to look at breast tissue. The purpose of a mammogram is to pick up early breast cancers before the tumor can be felt on an exam. It is believed that by the time a breast cancer is the size of a pea, it has already been present in the breast from three to seven *years*. Mammography can find many breast cancers before either you or your doctor can feel them. Detecting a breast cancer at this early stage will give you the best chance for a cure with the least amount of surgery.

How often should I get a mammogram?

Several years ago, routine mammography was reserved for women at high risk. During the last ten years the radiation exposure during mammography has been cut in half. Because the newer mammogram machines give a much clearer reading of breast tissue at half the radiation dose, the procedure has been advised for routine use in all women. The American Cancer Society has a number of suggestions.

- **All women should get a baseline mammogram between the ages of 35-40.**
- **Over age 50, a mammogram should be done yearly.**
- **If you have a strong family history suggestive of hereditary breast cancer, mammograms should be done as early as age 25, as discussed earlier.**

There is some controversy regarding how often mammograms should be performed between the ages of 40-50. Every year to once every three years has been suggested. Every two years seems a good compromise.

I've heard of other screening methods for breast cancer. What are they, and are they useful?

Over the years different screening methods have been tried, but none have been shown to be better than mammography. *Ultrasound, thermography,* and *transillumination* techniques of the breast have been studied by various investigators but their ability to pick up subclinical lesions is not sufficiently accurate to warrant their use as a sole screening procedure. Two techniques that may have some promise for the future are *digital radiography* and *magnetic resonance imaging* (MRI). Both of these procedures pose almost no radiation risk. They are considered experimental techniques at present, as their use is being further modified to apply to the breast. Expense may be a consideration in their use, as well.

Are mammograms painful?

Most women say that a mammogram is not painful, but it can be uncomfortable, especially if your breasts are tender. The examination should be performed when your breasts are the least tender to lessen your discomfort.

Underarm deodorants should not be used on the day of the exam because the *aluminum chloride* in many of the deodorants can create inaccurate images on the mammogram.

How accurate are mammograms in detecting early breast cancer?

Although mammography is very sensitive, it does not detect all cancers. There is about a 8-10% false-negative rate: a tumor can be felt on exam but the mammogram report is negative. *Any persistent clinically suspicious lump should be biopsied despite the mammogram report.*

If I have a suspicious mammogram, does it mean I have breast cancer?

No, it does not. Physicians look for suspicious *clustered microcalcifications* on a mammogram. These are very small (less than 1mm.) and represent calcium deposits within the breast that may be a sign of early breast cancer. All microcalcifications are not malignant, however. But if they are suspicious, they must be removed because 10% to 30% of microcalcifications turn out to be cancerous.

Has routine mammography increased the number of breast biopsies being performed?

Yes, it has increased the number of biopsies because most suspicious findings on mammography lead to a biopsy. Even though most of the biopsies are benign, mammography detects a significant number of breast cancers at the earliest stage. Mammography has also affected the work of the pathologists who read the biopsies under the microscope. They have had to learn about a number of new precancerous conditions of the breast that were not appreciated previously.

I've heard there is less surgery being performed for breast cancer. Is this true?

Recent studies have shown that having a "lumpectomy" and *axillary node dissection* to rule out metastases to the lymph nodes, followed by post operative radiation to prevent local recurrence has the same survival rate as the previously performed modified radical mastectomies (the removal of the entire breast and lymph nodes in one block of tissue). It is not the purpose of this discussion to go into the pros and cons of the various treatments of breast cancer, but you should know all your alternatives prior to deciding on the best treatment for you. Several states have now passed laws that require physicians to discuss with you all the alternatives to breast cancer surgery prior to deciding on your course of treatment.

12

What If I Need Surgery?

Since six of the ten most common surgeries performed in the United States are on the female reproductive system, there is a good chance that you will need or have already had some type of "female surgery." These include biopsies of the breast and uterus, D & C, Cesarean section, hysterectomy, tubal ligation, and ovarian cyst surgery. You may feel apprehensive and confused about the surgeries you may need during the menopausal period. Misperceptions abound. Often patients tell me that they have had a hysterectomy, yet they don't really know what was removed.

Nobody likes to face the possibility of surgery, but often it is essential in providing the best medical care for you. In this chapter, I will discuss the gynecologic surgical procedures that you are most likely to encounter during your menopausal years and alternatives to surgery, should any exist. I will also discuss several newer surgical techniques that are presently being perfected, including "laser hysterectomy" and the expanded laparoscopy procedures that will become more popular during the next few years.

DIAGNOSTIC PROCEDURES THAT SAMPLE THE ENDOMETRIUM

What is a biopsy?

During a biopsy, your physician removes a piece of tissue and examines it, usuallly under a microscope, in order to make a diagnosis. A breast biopsy is the removal and analysis of a piece of breast tissue, an endometrial biopsy studies tissue from the endometrium (uterine lining).

What is endometrial sampling?

In the years preceding your last period, or if you are on estrogen replacement therapy, it is not unusual to develop unexpected uterine bleeding. Your doctor may want to "sample" your uterine lining to make sure that nothing serious is causing the abnormal bleeding. An endometrial sampling can be done by an endometrial biopsy, an endometrial aspiration or a D & C. Any persistent abnormal uterine bleeding should be investigated by one of these sampling techniques.

What is an endometrial biopsy?

An endometrial biopsy is performed by passing a small, thin tube through the cervix and into the uterine cavity. As the tube is withdrawn, it scrapes against the uterine lining, trapping several small pieces of tissue within. This procedure is often performed as part of an infertility evaluation to determine if a woman is ovulating. It is also performed in cases of abnormal uterine bleeding in peri- and postmenopausal women. Recently developed small, thin tubes (as shown on page 199) make biopsies less painful than in the past.

What is an endometrial aspiration?

During an endometrial aspiration, a small thin tube is also passed through the cervix into the uterine cavity. The tube is attached to a syringe or suction machine that acts like a vacuum cleaner. It suctions or *aspirates* the uterine lining. An endometrial aspiration usually removes more tissue than an endometrial biopsy.

What is a D & C?

D & C stands for dilation and curettage. It is a surgical procedure in which the cervical opening is gradually made larger with *dilators* (a series of instruments that increase in size to widen an opening) to allow a spoon-shaped instrument, a *curette*, into the uterus to scrape and remove tissue. Your doctor performs a D & C as a diagnostic tool and as a form of treatment in certain diseases of the uterus. He can use it to treat incomplete miscarriages, where the remaining pregnancy tissue is removed. A D & C can also help diagnose and treat unexplained uterine bleeding during the menopausal period. (See illustration on page 200.)

Figure 12-1

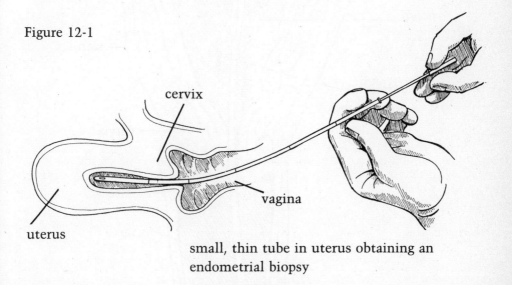

small, thin tube in uterus obtaining an endometrial biopsy

Endometrial biopsy.

What is the difference between an endometrial biopsy, endometrial aspiration, and D & C?

These procedures are all ways to obtain samples of the uterine lining for diagnosis. They offer varying degrees of completeness, and each has its place in the evaluation and treatment of abnormal bleeding. For an evaluation of the status of the uterine lining, a biopsy will suffice. For a removal of the uterine lining, an aspiration or D & C will be necessary.

Figure 12-2

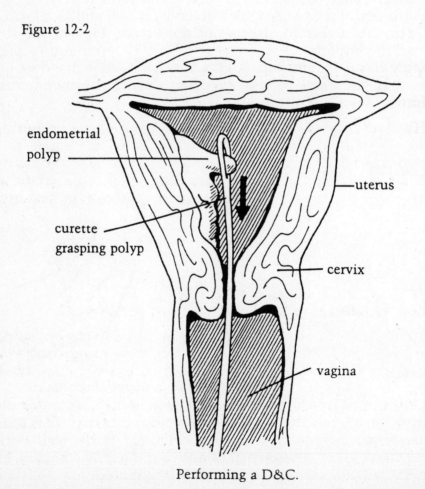

endometrial polyp

curette grasping polyp

uterus

cervix

vagina

Performing a D&C.

Are there other, noninvasive techniques used to evaluate the uterine lining?

Recently, as an alternative to endometrial biopsies, vaginal ultrasound examinations have been used to measure the thickness of the uterine lining in the menopausal women who are on hormonal therapy. If the endometrial thickness is 5mm or less, no hyperplasia or precancerous condition exists. If it measures greater than 5mm, an endometrial biopsy should be performed.

HYSTEROSCOPY

What is hysteroscopy?

Hysteroscopy is one of the "scoping" procedures becoming more popular in gynecologic surgery. A hysteroscope is a narrow light-containing telescope inserted through the cervix that allows your physician to look directly into the uterus at the uterine lining for both diagnostic and surgical procedures.

Where is a hysteroscopy examination performed?

Most gynecologists perform this procedure in the operating room of a hospital or surgery center. Office hysteroscopy is becoming more popular as better equipment becomes available.

During hysteroscopy, a liquid solution or carbon dioxide gas is introduced into the uterus to distend the cavity. This may cause some cramps but may be tolerated fairly well with local anesthesia. A biopsy or endometrial aspiration may be performed after the hysteroscopy is completed.

How does hysteroscopy differ from a D & C?

Hysteroscopy allows a direct look at the entire uterine lining. On the other hand, your doctor performs a D & C by scraping a curette inside the uterine cavity without looking directly within. A D & C is a "blind" procedure in the sense that the physician does not see what is being scraped. Often, even the best of surgeons can leave a large area of the uterine lining untouched despite a "complete scraping." It is not unusual to miss small submucous fibroids (fibroids protruding into the uterine cavity) during a D & C. These can be visualized at the time of a hysteroscopy examination.

Is hysteroscopy better than a D & C?

Hysteroscopy has gained in popularity in recent years as a more direct method of diagnosing abnormal uterine bleeding. It is possible to pass over polyps or submucous fibroids during a D & C. With hysteroscopy, physicians have a direct view of the uterine lining. They need no longer depend on how the cavity "feels." The combination of hysteroscopy with one of the various laser or electrosurgical instruments to ablate, or destroy, the uterine lining is becoming an alternative to hysterectomy for the treatment of certain types of abnormal uterine bleeding.

HYSTERECTOMY

What is a hysterectomy?

The word hysterectomy is derived from the Greek words *hyster,* meaning uterus and *ectomy* for removal. Hysterectomy is the surgical removal of the uterus.

What is a total hysterectomy?

A *total hysterectomy* is the removal of both the corpus (body) and the cervix (mouth or neck) of the uterus. Years ago, when surgical and anesthetic techniques were not as sophisticated as today, only the body of the uterus was removed. The cervix was often left behind. This is referred to as a *subtotal hysterectomy*. Today when a woman states she had a "total" hysterectomy, she often means her uterus, tubes, and ovaries were removed. Technically this is incorrect. She actually had a hysterectomy with a *bilateral salpingoophorectomy* (removal of the uterus, both tubes, and both ovaries).

What is a oophorectomy?

Oophoros is Greek for ovary. *Oophorectomy* is the surgical removal of the ovary. A *unilateral oophorectomy* means one ovary was taken; a *bilateral oophorectomy* means both were removed.

What is a *salpingectomy*?

Salpinx is Greek for tube. A *salpingectomy* is the surgical removal of the Fallopian tube. A *unilateral salpingectomy* means one Fallopian tube was taken; a *bilateral salpingectomy* means both were taken.

What is a *salpingoophorectomy*?

This is the removal of a Fallopian tube and an ovary. Again, if one side is removed, the procedure is designated a *unilateral salpingoophorectomy*, and if both sides are taken, it's a *bilateral sapingoophorectomy*.

How is a hysterectomy performed?

A hysterectomy may be performed in one of two ways; through the abdomen (an *abdominal hysterectomy*) or through the vagina (a *vaginal hysterectomy*). Each has its advantages and disadvantages. It will be up to your surgeon, after discussing the alternatives with you, to decide which will be the best for you. Most gynecologic surgeons (and patients) prefer the vaginal hysterectomy, if at all possible. The operating time and recovery period are shorter, and the woman usually experiences less post-operative discomfort.

What are the advantages of a vaginal hysterectomy?

The advantages of a vaginal hysterectomy include:

- **no visible scar on the abodomen**
- **less operating and anesthesia time**
- **shorter hospital stay and recovery time**
- **less chance of gas pains and adhesion formation**
- **less post-operative pain**

In addition, a cystocele or rectocele repair can be performed at the same time as the hysterectomy without repositioning you on the operating table. This markedly reduces the operating time.

What are the disadvantages of a vaginal hysterectomy?

The disadvantages of a vaginal hysterectomy are as follows.

- **The uterus must be of normal size or just slightly enlarged or else it cannot be removed through the vagina.**
- **The surgeon cannot explore the remainder of the abdominal cavity or be assured of removing the ovaries if needed.**
- **The incidence of post-operative infection is slightly higher than in an abdominal hysterectomy.**

What different types of incisions can be performed with an abdominal hysterectomy?

There are two types of incisions: a vertical (up and down) incision going from just above your pubic bone to just below or next to your bellybutton (umbilicus) and the so-called "bikini incision" or *Plannensteil* incision. It goes parallel to and at the approximate level of your pubic hair line. It is a transverse incision and is covered if a bikini bathing suit is worn.

What are the advantages of each of these incisions?

The type of incision your doctor recommends may simply depend on habit. Some surgeons get used to one type of incision and do want to vary their technique. If you have a very large pelvic mass or a suspected malignancy, you are better off with a vertical incision, as it gives more exposure at the time of surgery and allows your physician to explore the entire abdominal cavity. With a bikini incision, there is less room to operate. It is very difficult to explore the upper abdominal cavity (the liver, stomach, and gallbladder area) if necessary. The advantage of the bikini incision is that it heals with a much thinner scar and is less visible.

How long is the recovery time following a hysterectomy?

The hospital stay following surgery is getting shorter each year. Presently, most patients are hospitalized for between three and five days following a hysterectomy. They are absent from work on average of four to six weeks. Frequent bending and heavy lifting should be avoided for six weeks. Even though you may be back to feeling fairly well by this time, it is not unusual to have some lingering discomfort and tiredness for an additional two to four weeks. Some women state they don't feel they have returned to normal for approximately six months following their surgery. The recovery time for a vaginal hysterectomy is usually shorter compared with that for an abdominal hysterectomy.

When is a hysterectomy indicated?

The removal of the uterus is indicated for one of several different conditions. These include:

- large fibroid tumors
- endometriosis
- pelvic relaxation, such as a prolapsed uterus, cystocele, enterocele, or rectocele
- severe dysmenorrhea (painful periods) not controllable by more conservative measures
- chronic pelvic infections
- persistent abnormal uterine bleeding not helped by a D & C
- cancers of the cervix, endometrium, tubes, or ovaries

I've heard a lot about unnecessary hysterectomies. Are there alternatives to a hysterectomy?

Most hysterectomies performed in this country are for nonlife-threatening conditions. Depending on the severity and symptoms you have prior to your contemplated surgery, you may elect to try alternatives. If you are experiencing recurrent dysfunctional uterine bleeding (abnormal uterine bleeding with no apparent cause and thought to be hormonal), a several month trial of cyclic hormonal therapy with a progestational agent or an estrogen-progesterone regimen may be indicated. All fibroid tumors do not have to be removed. If they are small, not causing abnormal uterine bleeding, and do not suddenly grow, they can be followed until menopause occurs, at which time the fiboird should become smaller. An estrogen-dependent fibroid should go away after you stop menstruating. If you are experiencing heavy menstrual periods that do not respond to other conservative measures, and you do not want a hysterectomy, you can undergo a procedure called laser ablation of the uterine lining.

LASER SURGERY AND ELECTROSURGERY

What are laser surgery and electrosurgery?

In these types of surgery, a source of energy is directed through a fiber-optic endoscope (a telescope-type instrument that is used for looking inside an organ or body cavity) to cut or cauterize tissue. Examples of operating endoscopes are the cystoscope, to look inside the bladder; the hysteroscope, to look inside the uterine cavity; and the laparoscope, to look inside the abdominal cavity at the pelvic organs. Laser surgery uses a laser beam as its energy source. Among the types of lasers used in gynecological surgery today are the carbon dioxide, argon, KTP, and YAG lasers. Each has different characteristics and is used for different surgical procedures.

Electrosurgery uses an electric current as its energy source. Advancements in laser, electrical, and laparascopic equipment have made both types of surgery safer and easier to perform.

What is laser ablation of the uterine lining?

Laser ablation is the use of a laser beam directed through a hysteroscope to abolish and destroy the uterine lining. It has chiefly been used in woman who are having extremely heavy menstrual periods that are not helped by some of the more conservative measures described in Chapter 3.

How is laser ablation of the uterine lining performed?

Your doctor inserts a hysteroscope through the cervix and directs a laser beam through the scope to destroy the entire uterine lining. The beam penetrates as deeply as the muscle layer so the lining will not regenerate. Laser ablation is becoming more popular as more gynecologists are trained in the technique. Although the procedure has been referred to as a "laser hysterectomy," it is not a hysterectomy, but may be a viable alternative to that surgery in certain instances. Small submucous fibroids and polyps may also be treated with the laser through the hysteroscope.

What are the advantages of laser ablation of the uterine lining?

Laser ablation can be performed in a one-day surgery center with little discomfort or recuperation needed before resuming normal activity. The recovery time may only be a few days, compared to six to eight weeks for a hysterectomy. It may be a good alternative if the abnormal bleeding you are experiencing meets the criteria to have the surgery performed and a hysterectomy is your only other option.

What are the disadvantages of laser ablation of the uterine lining?

Presently, there are only a few trained laser surgeons, and the equipment is very expensive. Laser ablation is not available in every area of the country. Since this is a relatively new procedure, long-term follow-up on patients is still under way. The preliminary data on the procedure, however, show no major problems, and a good rate of success. Yet it is still uncertain what will happen to the uterine lining of women who have undergone the procedure, should they need estrogen replacement at the time of menopause. If the entire lining is destroyed and does not regenerate, estrogen therapy should not have an effect on the uterus.

What is a "Roller-Ball Hysterectomy"?

This is a method of electrosurgery, similar to a laser ablation, that is used to ablate, or destroy, the uterine lining. A medical device called an resectoscope is inserted through the hysteroscope; the doctor can thus see inside the uterus while he is performing the procedure. The resectoscope has an attachment on the end that destroys the uterine lining and submucous fibroids by either shaving them with a thin razor edge or cauterizing them with a roller-ball-tipped probe.

LAPAROSCOPY

What is a laparoscopy examination?

Laparoscopy is the use of a light-containing telescope which is placed through the abdomen at the level of the naval (umbilicus) to look directly at the pelvic organs. Laparoscopy is used both for diagnostic and treatment purposes. It is often referred to as "band-aid" or "bellybutton" surgery. The gynecologist has a direct look at the pelvic organs to rule out abnormalities, such as adhesions or endometriosis.

When is laparoscopy indicated?

Laparoscopy is used:

- **in evaluating the infertile female**
- **in evaluating severe pelvic pain**
- **in diagnosing the origins of severe menstrual cramps**
- **in diagnosing pelvic masses or ovarian cysts**
- **to perform what used to be considered major surgery**

A laparoscopic tubal ligation is the most common form of sterilization. In addition, laser beam or electrosurgical current can also be directed through a laparoscope to destroy endometriosis implants and even remove small ectopic pregnancies.

Figure 12-3

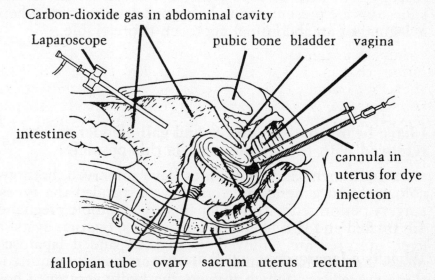

Carbon-dioxide gas in abdominal cavity

Laparoscope · · · pubic bone · bladder · vagina

intestines

cannula in uterus for dye injection

fallopian tube · ovary · sacrum · uterus · rectum

Laparoscopy with woman lying on her back.

Is laparoscopy major surgery?

Laparoscopy is considered minor surgery, but most of the time it requires a general anesthetic. This procedure is usually performed on an out-patient basis in a one-day surgery center, but occasionally an overnight stay may be necessary. If a problem is found at the time of a laparoscopy exam that cannot be treated through the laparoscope, major surgery with an abdominal incision, may be performed.

How is laparoscopy most commonly used in the perimenopausal woman?

This procedure is most commonly used in women over 40 for sterilization purposes. Your physician may also rely on it if he feels a pelvic mass and cannot tell whether it is an ovarian cyst or a fibroid tumor of the uterus. With laparoscopy, he can have a direct look at the pelvic organs. Laparoscopy may also be used prior to a hysterectomy to see if adhesions are present and to help your doctor decide whether a vaginal or an abdominal approach is preferable.

I have heard that the uterus and gall bladder can be removed with the laparoscope. Is this possible?

As equipment and techniques have improved, both gynecological and general surgeons have expanded the types of surgery performed with the laparoscope. Ectopic pregnancies are treated and gall bladders, appendices, ovarian cysts, and even uteruses are removed through expanded laparoscopy procedures. Multiple small incisions are usually required for these procedures, which involve markedly shortened hospital stays and recovery times.

What are the advantages of the expanded laparoscopy procedures?

The hospitalization and recovery time from a laparoscopy procedure are much shorter than a major abdominal procedure. An overnight hospitalization may be all that is necessary, compared with three to six days for a *laparotomy* (an operation requiring an abdominal incision). Laparoscopy equipment is not available in all hospitals, and the surgeons utilizing the equipment must have special training.

CONDITIONS THAT REQUIRE SURGERY: A MASS ON THE OVARY

What is an ovarian cyst?

A cyst is any sac which contains a liquid or semisolid substance. An ovarian cyst grows within the ovary. Ovarian cysts are either functional or pathologic.

What are functional ovarian cysts?

Functional ovarian cysts are related to the normal function of the ovary. They may be *follicular* (a cyst of the *Graafian follicle* present before ovulation) or *luteal*. The latter may form after ovulation and is related to the *corpus luteum*. (See Chapter 2.) Most functional cysts will not become larger than 5–6cm. (the size of a large egg), but occasionally they do grow beyond this size.

Are functional cysts more common during the perimenopausal years?

Unfortunately, they are. If you start having irregular cycles prior to menopause, your hormones are being produced in an uneven manner. This causes sporadic ovulation. A follicular cyst may develop and become very large (the size of an orange or grapefruit). Occasionally, after you ovulate, the corpus luteum becomes very large, as well.

What are pathologic ovarian cysts?

Pathologic ovarian cysts are related to abnormal growths of one of the cells within the ovary. They may be either benign (non-cancerous) or malignant (cancerous). Common benign pathologic cysts are *dermoid cysts, serous cystadenomas, mucinous cystadenomas, fibromas, cystadenofibromas,* and *endometrioma* (an ovarian cyst containing endometriosis). The two most common malignant ovarian cysts are *serous cystadenocarcinomas* and *mucinous cystadenocarcinomas.* Pathologic ovarian cysts are usually larger than the functional cysts, but they all start off small. Just because a cyst is small is no guarantee that it is benign.

Do ovarian cysts create symptoms?

Small ovarian cysts will not be symptomatic. If a cyst becomes large it may cause:

- **pressure feeling in the pelvis**
- **abdominal or pelvic pain**
- **pressure on the bladder causing urinary frequency**
- **constipation with pressure on the rectum**
- **irregular menstrual periods**

A cyst may twist on itself (called *torsion*) causing extreme pain. Or it may burst, spilling its contents into the abdominal cavity, also causing sudden and marked abdominal pain. (This is occasionally seen with a ruptured endometriosis cyst.) These two conditions may require emergency surgery.

How are ovarian cysts diagnosed?

Most are diagnosed during an annual pelvic exam. If there is a question as to the size or exact location of the cyst, further investigational studies such as an ultrasound, CT scan, or laparoscopy may be necessary. Although these may show how large the cyst is, they usually cannot give an exact diagnosis, such as whether it is benign or malignant. A blood test known as Ca-125 may differentiate between benign and malignant ovarian cysts.

What is the treatment of an ovarian cyst?

Functional ovarian cysts will go away by themselves. If your doctor suspects the cyst is functional, he may have you come back after you finish your next menstrual period to recheck its size, at which time a functional cyst would be much smaller or even gone. Often birth control pills are prescribed for a few months to "suppress" ovulation and help shrink a functional cysts. If a cyst persists beyond this period of time, surgery may be necessary to remove it, or the ovary itself, for an exact diagnosis and treatment.

What if the cyst is found to be malignant?

The preferred treatment for a malignant ovarian cyst in the perimenopausal woman is a total hysterectomy with a bilateral salpingoophorectomy (complete removal of the uterus, tubes, and ovaries). If you still desire children, it may be possible to preserve the uterus and one ovary with certain types of ovarian malignancies. Sampling of other intra-abdominal tissues such as the peritoneal fluid, omentum, and lymph nodes is often performed at the time of surgery if a malignancy is found.

Why is it necessary to remove the uterus and other ovary if only one ovary is involved with cancer?

The uterus, tubes, and ovaries share a common blood supply and lymphatic drainage. If one ovary is cancerous, the other organs are also removed in case the cancer has spread microscopically to the uterus or other ovary.

What is the significance of an enlarged ovary in a postmenopausal woman?

Once you have stopped menstruating, your ovaries have stopped working and should not develop functional cysts. Any ovarian cyst that forms in a postmenopausal woman is presumed to be pathologic with the possibility of cancer being present. Therefore, a cyst in a postmenopausal woman should be looked at and removed for further diagnosis and treatment. Often cancer of the ovary cannot be diagnosed until the ovary is examined under the microscope. This, of course, requires its removal. An ultrasound examination and a Ca-125 blood test may help in evaluating the ovary to decide if surgery is necessary.

ABNORMAL PAP SMEARS AND CERVICAL CANCER

What is colposcopy?

Colpos is a Greek word which refers to the vagina. *Colposcopy* is a procedure which utilizes an operating microscope to look at the cervix and vagina. It helps magnify and identify the origin of abnormal cells detected on a Pap smear. A small biopsy can be taken of any suspicious lesions.

Where is colposcopy performed?

Colposcopy is usually performed wherever a colposcope is available. Many gynecologists have this instrument in their offices or have access to one in the out-patient department of their hospitals. Colposcopy is performed in much the same way as a pelvic examination. Usually no special anesthetic or preparation is needed. If your gynecologist detects a suspicious area through the colposcope, she will take a small biopsy, and send it to the pathologist for microscopic examination. The use of colposcopy and biopsies has eliminated many of the cervical conizations that were performed in the past for the evaluation of abnormal pap smears.

What is a *cervical* conization?

This is a surgical procedure in which an ice cream cone shaped piece of tissue is removed from the center of the uterine cervix for the diangosis and treatment of abnormal pap smears. If, on evaluation with colposcopy, suspicious cells are found going into the endocervical canal (the canal leading from the external cervix to the beginning of the uterine cavity), a conization may have to be performed to remove a portion of the canal. Cervical conizations are also performed if a colposcopy exam (after an abnormal pap smear) is inconclusive. It can be used to treat certain *dysplasias* and *carcinoma in situ* of the cervix. Laser surgery also can be used to perform cervical conizations.

Where is a cervical conization performed?

Most conizations are performed in a hospital operating room or surgery center. A recently developed electrosurgical conization called a LEEP (loop electrical excision procedure) can be performed in an office setting if the proper equipment is available.

What is cryosurgery?

Cryosurgery is a freezing technique usually applied to the external part of the cervix to treat abnormal cells found at the time of colposcopy. It is one of the ways to treat different abnormal conditions of the cervix (various degrees of *dysplasia* or *carcinoma-in-situ*.) Cryosurgery is usually performed in the office and results in only minimal cramping.

STERILIZATION

What is a tubal ligation?

During a tubal ligation or tubal sterilization procedure, the Fallopian tubes are cut, cauterized, clipped, banded, or partially removed for the purpose of preventing further pregnancies.

How is a tubal ligation performed?

A tubal ligation is usually performed by the way of laparoscopy on an out-patient basis. Sterilization can also be performed at the time of abdominal surgery, such as a C-section, or following a vaginal delivery by making a small one-half to one inch umbilical incision. A general anesthestic is usually required, although some physicians may perform these under local anesthesia.

PELVIC RELAXATION

What is pelvic relaxation?

This is a term used to describe a group of conditions related to a weakening and loss of support of the ligaments and structures around the uterus, bladder, vagina, and rectum. Uterine prolapse, cystoceles with or without stress incontinence, enteroceles, and rectoceles are all part of the pelvic relaxation syndromes which were discussed in detail in Chapter 6.

What type of surgery is performed for the pelvic relaxation syndromes?

The most common surgical procedure is a vaginal hysterectomy, a cystocele, and a rectocele repair. The latter are also called an anterior-posterior repair because of their location with respect to the vagina. Even if you do not have a significant degree of uterine prolapse, the uterus is best removed at the time of a bladder repair, so it woll not pull and loosen the stitches holding the bladder in place following surgery. The success rate of the surgery is greater if the uterus is removed at the same time as the bladder repair than if it were left in place. If you still desire children, however, the bladder can be repaired without disturbing the uterus.

How is an anterior-posterior repair performed?

Most of the time this surgery is performed through the vagina. The uterus is removed and then the cystocele and rectocele are repaired. A general anesthetic is usually used, but it can be performed with spinal anesthetic so that you remain awake.

How successful is pelvic relaxation surgery?

Surgery for stress incontinence has an approximate 85% success rate. If you have a chronic cough from bronchitis or are obese, the chances of recurrence will be greater because of the increase in intra-abdominal pressure on your pelvis following surgery.

What if my symptoms recur following surgery?

In about 10%-15% of cases, there can be a recurrence of symptoms from a few months to (more commonly) a few years after surgery. Several surgical procedures suspending the bladder through an abdominal approach are utilized for the treatment of recurrent stress incontinence. Several newer operations use sling type sutures, suspending the bladder with very small incisions. This type of surgery requires very little time in the hospital.

I am going to have an abdominal hysterectomy because of large fibroids. I also have stress incontinence. Can my doctor perform both surgeries at once?

If you are having an abdominal hysterectomy, you can have a Marshall-Marchetti operation at the same time. This operation utilizes stitches to support the urethral-vesicular angle (the angle between the urethra and bladder) to the pubic bone through the same abdominal incision as the hysterectomy. Some surgeons prefer this approach. If a large cystocele is present, however, a vaginal approach will be necessary. Occasionally, a combined vaginal and abdominal approach is utilized to obtain the best results.

After having several children, I feel "loose" with intercourse. Can anything be done to tighten my muscles?

It is not unusual for your vaginal opening to become loose after bearing children. Some looseness does not interfere with satisfactory sexual relations. You may wish to try Kegel exercises to tighten the muscles around the vagina and rectum.

(See Chapter 6.) If this is unsuccessful, an operation called a *perineorrhaphy* or *perineoplasty* can be performed.

What is a perineorrhaphy and perineoplasty?

In this operation, excess skin and vaginal tissue are removed from the entrance to the vagina and stitches are utilized to tighten the vaginal opening. Often, a perineorrhaphy can be combined with a vaginal hysterectomy and bladder or rectocele repair if you discuss this option with your doctor before surgery.

13

Should I Take Hormone Replacement?

Once you've gone through menopause, you may want to consider whether or not you should start estrogen replacement therapy. Every woman is different, and your symptoms should be evaluated and treated on an individual basis. You will live more than one-third of your life after menopause, so the postmenopausal years should be as enjoyable as possible. Many times, estrogen therapy can make a difference between living a good life or simply existing. You and your physician should jointly decide whether or not you should take estrogen.

This book is not intended to replace your physician's advice, but rather to enable you to be more knowledgeable and capable of discussing with your physician your concerns about estrogen replacement therapy. In this chapter, I will summarize the advantages and disadvantages of estrogen replacement therapy, whether progesterone should be added to the treatment program, the different ways to take estrogen, and the types of estrogen and progesterone available.

ADVANTAGES AND DISADVANTAGES OF ESTROGEN REPLACEMENT THERAPY

What are the advantages of estrogen replacement therapy?

Estrogen therapy has been successful in reversing and/or preventing the physiological changes that occur after menopause. These include:

- hot flashes
- urogenital atrophy (vaginal dryness, painful intercourse, urinary urgency, and incontinence)
- wrinkling of the skin
- sleep disturbances
- mood changes, anxiety, and depression

Other important health benefits include the prevention of osteoporosis, a positive effect on cholesterol metabolism and a lower incidence of heart attacks. If a degenerative musculoskeletal disorderm such as rheumatoid arthritis, worsens after menopause, estrogen may also be beneficial.

What are the disadvantages of estrogen replacement therapy?

The disadvantages of estrogen replacement therapy include:

- nausea
- headache
- breast tenderness
- fluid retention
- depression
- breakthrough bleeding
- slight increase in incidence of gallstones

If a progestin is also prescribed as part of your therapy, the possible side effects include:

- **abdominal bloating**
- **headaches**
- **breast pain**
- **nervousness**
- **continuation of menstrual bleeding**

If you are on estrogen therapy and develop uterine bleeding unrelated to withdrawal bleeding from the progestin, your doctor may require an endometrial aspiration or a D & C, thus increasing the possibilities of the need for investigational studies and minor surgical procedures.

Why has there been so much controversy over estrogen replacement therapy?

The use of estrogen in postmenopausal women has gone through three different cycles over the last 30 years. The first cycle occurred during the 1960s, when several researchers and prominent physicians emphasized the benefits of estrogen therapy during the postmenopausal years. As a result, estrogen therapy became very popular. As complications became evident in the late 1970s and early 1980s, the second cycle started. Both physicians and patients became fearful of estrogen. Presently, there is a trend back toward estrogen replacement, as the benefits appear to outweigh the potential risks if estrogen is prescribed in an appropriate manner. This swinging of the estrogen pendulum has led to controversy and confusion about estrogen replacement therapy.

What influenced the trend against estrogen replacement during the 1970s and early 1980s?

Postmenopausal women on unopposed estrogen replacement therapy (estrogen without the progestin) started developing hyperplasia and cancer of the uterine lining. Studies showed that if a woman used estrogen for more than five years, she had a definite risk of developing cancer of the endometrium (uterine lining) if a progestin was not added to the regimen. The DES story connecting embryonic and fetal exposure of DES to cervical *adenosis, clearcell adenocarcinoma* of the vagina and defects in the female and male reproductive system, also frightened many people.

What is DES?

DES is an abbreviation for *diethylstilbesterol*, a synthetic estrogen that was commonly administered during the 1950s and 1960s to prevent miscarriages in pregnant women who were bleeding in the first several months of their pregnancy. Not only did it fail to prevent miscarriages, but it was later found to have serious side effects, including abnormalities of the female and male reproductive systems in children of the women who had taken DES.

Did the use of oral contraceptives (birth control pill) have an influence on whether estrogen was prescribed?

Studies about the side effects of the birth control pill, which contains a larger amount and different type of estrogen and progestin than used in postmenopausal therapy, also deterred physicians and the public from using estrogen replacement. The incidence of *thrombophlebitis*, strokes, and heart attacks with the higher dose birth control pills was perceived to apply to postmenopausal estrogen replacement, as well. As a result, physicians were very reluctant to prescribe estrogen and patients were very hesitant to take it for a number of years.

What influenced physicians back toward estrogen replacement therapy?

Research data showed that the addition of a progestational agent to both cyclic and continuous estrogen therapy prevented the development of estrogen-induced endometrial hyperplasia and cancer. In fact, the incidence of these conditions was actually *lower* in women who took estrogen and progesterone than in women who were *never* on estrogen therapy. Estrogen-progestin therapy may actually protect against the development of endometrial hyperplasia and endometrial cancer. Evidence also started appearing in the medical literature that estrogen was beneficial in preventing osteoporosis and heart attacks.

Are there women who should not take estrogen?

Estrogen replacement therapy is not for all women. The reasons some women should not take estrogen are usually separated into absolute and relative contraindications. Those who absolutely cannot take estrogen are women with:

- **a previously diagnosed or suspected breast cancer**
- **active liver disease**
- **active *thrombophlebitis* (blood clots)**
- ***thromboembolic* disorders (the release of clots which go to the brain causing small strokes).**

What are the relative contraindications?

A relative contraindication is one in which estrogen therapy would not generally be used unless the benefit far exceeds the potential risks. These include women with:

- **chronic liver disorders**
- **marked obesity**
- **pre-existing uterine myomas (fibroids)**
- **a history of thrombophlebitis or thromboembolism**
- **a history of endometriosis**
- **a past history of endometrial cancer.**

Some of these relative contraindications are of more concern than others. If you are on estrogen with any of these conditions, you should be monitored closely by your physician. The route of administration of estrogen may also be of importance in some cases of relative contraindications, as they are related to how estrogen is metabolized by the liver.

LIVER METABOLISM

Why should I be concerned about the liver?

The liver plays a role in the way estrogen may be administered. Many of the side effects and contraindications of estrogen therapy are influenced by their effect on the liver.

What is the function of the liver?

The liver is a large organ located in the right upper quadrant of the abdominal cavity. It is essential for life. The liver serves many functions:

- **converting and storing the sugars we ingest in the form of glycogen**
- **manufacturing cholesterol which is used by the various endocrine glands to make hormones**
- **producing bile which helps in fat absorption**
- **producing many essential proteins we utilize for the normal functioning of our body.**

The proteins related to estrogen therapy include:

- **proteins that carry the hormones from one place to another in our bodies**
- **protein-clotting factors that make our blood coagulate in order to stop unwanted bleeding**
- **proteins responsible for stabilization of blood pressure**
- **proteins that transport the lipids from one place to another in our bodies.**

Where does the liver get its nourishment and blood supply?

The liver receives its blood from two large vessels. The first is the *hepatic artery* which comes from the aorta and supplies oxygenated blood and nutrients from the general circulation to the liver. The other is the *portal vein* which comes from the stomach and intestinal tract. All the food and medication we consume gets absorbed by the stomach and intestines and goes to the liver by way of the portal vein before it enters into the general circulation.

ESTROGEN METABOLISM AND THE LIVER

How does the portal vein system work with regard to estrogen replacement therapy?

The portal vein blood supply to the liver is often referred to as the *entero-hepatic* (intestinal-liver) circulation. In reference to estrogen therapy, the entero-hepatic circulation is called the first pass of estrogen through the liver.

After estrogens given orally enter the liver where they become metabolized to a less active form, they then enter the general circulation where they exert their influence on the other organs. Estrogen in the portal vein is four to five times more concentrated than in the general circulation. It is for this reason that an equal dose of estrogen given orally has a greater effect on the liver than estrogens given by injection, vaginal route, or skin patch. With the non-oral methods of administration, estrogen enters the general circulation first, and only later enters the liver via the hepatic artery, and then in a less concentrated dose.

What liver proteins are affected by estrogen?

Estrogen stimulates the production of many of the proteins manufactured by the liver which transfer the various hormones in our body. The *sex hormone-binding globulin* (a type of protein), *cortisol-binding globulin, thyroid-binding globulin, iron-binding globulin,* and a *copper-binding protein* are all stimulated by estrogen therapy. The increase in these proteins has *no known* negative effect on your body but may alter the results of laboratory tests affecting these hormones if you are pregnant, on estrogen replacement therapy or on the birth control pill. This is why women taking any form of estrogen, or who are pregnant, have altered thyroid function tests, yet continue to have normal thyroid function. Certain thyroid tests measure the protein binding in the thyroid hormone which is elevated during pregnancy and in women on estrogen medications. In order for your physician to interpret these tests, she should know if you are taking estrogen or any other medication.

How does estrogen affect blood pressure?

Estrogen may cause an increase in a liver protein called *renin substrate (angiotensinogen).* Angiotensinogen influences blood pressure by its effect on the *renin-angiotensin-aldosterone* (a liver-kidney connection) system, the body's blood pressure regulator. Some of the different estrogens stimulate the angiotensin system more than others. The synthetic estrogen *ethinyl estradiol* influences this blood pressure system to a greater degree than do the naturally occurring estrogens, which are more commonly used in postmenopausal estrogen therapy. This is why some women on birth control pills (which contain ethinyl estradiol) are susceptible to an increase in blood pressure. Women on estrogen replacement therapy, where natural estrogens are more commonly used, are less likely to experience an increase in blood pressure. In fact, most estrogens used in postmenopausal hormone therapy have been shown to lower blood pressure.

How does estrogen affect the clotting mechanism in our blood?

Estrogen may stimulate the production of some of the clotting factors produced by the liver. Again, the synthetic estrogen, ethinyl estradiol, has a much greater effect on the clotting factors than the natural estrogens. Birth control pills increase the risk of thromboembolic (both thrombophlebitis and embolism) disease whereas the natural estrogens do not. In fact, several studies have shown that *conjugated equine estrogen* (Premarin), used in the menopausal woman, does *not* affect the liver clotting proteins and clotting tendency. The effect on the clotting mechanism also accounts for the reduction of ethinyl estradiol from over 100mcg to 30-35mcg in the low-dose birth control pills during the last several years. The effect of estrogen on the clotting mechanism is related to the type, dosage, and the absorption route of the estrogen. (Estrogens which go through the liver first have the greatest effect.)

How does estrogen affect lipid metabolism?

Estrogen stimulates the liver's production of cholesterol, causing an increase in the HDL-cholesterol level, and a decrease in the LDL-cholesterol level, both of which help prevent heart attacks. The proteins that transfer the lipids from one place to another are also affected by estrogen. Chapter 9 discusses the influence of estrogen on lipid metabolism, and its relationship to cardiovascular disease in greater detail.

Does estrogen affect gallbladder disease?

The gallbladder is a sac located beneath the liver that stores the bile produced by the liver. Bile is needed to help digest fatty substances after they enter the small intestine. Women taking oral contraceptives and women on estrogen therapy have a two- to threefold increased risk of developing gallstones and gallbladder disease than women not on estrogen therapy. Estrogen increases the cholesterol fraction of bile which may result in stone formation. This slight increase in the risk of gallbladder disease is one of the negative factors of estrogen replacement therapy. Estrogen that does not first pass through the liver, such as the skin patch, will not have as great an effect on gallstones as an estrogen that does have a first pass through the liver, such as the pill.

Are the effects of estrogen on the liver good or bad?

It's a mixed blessing. Estrogen is bad in the sense that it may cause high blood pressure, an increase in clotting problems and gallbladder disease. But it is beneficial to lipid metabolism because it increases the HDL-cholesterol level and decreases the LDL-cholesterol level. I would like to emphasize, however, that the effect of estrogen on the liver depends on the type and amount of estrogen administered. The synthetic estrogens appear to stimulate the liver proteins to a much greater degree than the natural estrogens. If the effects of the natural estrogen on the liver are still a concern, they can be further reduced by avoiding oral estrogen entirely in favor of the skin patch, a vaginal cream, or the injectable preparations. The preparations that avoid the initial pass through the liver, however, will *not* be as beneficial to cholesterol metabolism as the oral estrogen. The effects on the liver of the synthetic estrogen ethinyl estradiol may be related more to its dosage than to its being synthetic. The dose of ethinyl estradiol that would be equivalent to the 0.625mg of conjugated estrogens is $5\mu g$, or one-fourth to one-seventh of the dose $(20–35\mu g)$ in the lowest-dose birth control pills.

TYPES OF ESTROGEN

What are the different types of estrogen?

There are two types of estrogen in general use: synthetic (made in a laboratory) estrogens and the naturally occurring estrogens normally found in your body.

What are the synthetic estrogens?

The synthetic estrogens are made by chemists in a laboratory. They consist of *ethinyl estradiol* and its derivatives. The oral forms of the synthetic estrogen include: *ethinyl estraiol* (Estinyl), *quinestrol* (Estrovis) and *diethylstilbestrol* (DES).

What are the oral forms of the naturally occurring estrogens?

The natural estrogens are identical to the estrogens normally found in the body. The oral forms of the natural estrogens include: *conjugated equine estrogen* (Premarin), *estrone sulfate* (Ogen), *esterified estrogens* (Estratab), *estradiol valerate* (Progynova) and *micronized estradiol* (Estrace). Generic preparations exist for many of these estrogens. (See Table 1.)

What is the difference between the synthetic and naturally occurring estrogens?

The synthetic estrogens are much more potent than the naturally occurring preparations. The synthetics, when taken orally, affect the liver proteins to a greater degree than do the natural estrogens, although this appears to be related to the dosage. The synthetic estrogens have been used principally in the birth control pill, where a more potent estrogen is needed to suppress ovulation. The natural estrogens will not suppress ovulation and are not used in oral contraceptives. Since the natural estrogens affect the liver proteins to a lesser degree than do the synthetics, the former are more commonly used in postmenopausal therapy. However, we may see very low doses of synthetic estrogens in future drug hormone replacement regimens.

Are the generic brands of estrogen as good as the brand names?

Over the last several years, the use of generic medications has increased. Some of the generic brands may be equivalent, but I personally have found (and studies have verified my suspicions) that the generic conjugated estrogens do not consistently relieve menopausal symptoms as well as the brand name of conjugated estrogens, Premarin. The generics may not contain the appropriate amount of medication, and they may be coated with a substance that is not absorbed well through the intestines. I prefer prescribing a brand name estrogen. I have had patients go to refill their brand name estrogen who have had a generic brand substituted without their

TABLE 1			
ORAL ESTROGENS			
BRAND NAME	GENERIC NAME	DOSAGE AVAILABLE IN MG	MANUFACTURER
Estinyl	Ethinyl Estradiol	.02, .05, .5	Schering
Estrace	Micronized Estradiol	1.0, 2.0	Mead Johnson
Estratab	Esterified Estrogens	0.3, 0.625, 1.25, 2.5	Solvay
Estrovis	Quinestrol	0.1	Parke-Davis
Ogen	Estropipate	0.625, 1.25, 2.5, 5.0	Abbott
Premarin	Conjugated Estrogens	0.3, 0.625, 0.9, 1.25, 2.5	Wyeth-Ayerst
Tace	Chlorotrianisene	12, 25, 72	Merrill-Dow

TABLE 2			
PARENTERAL ESTROGENS			
BRAND NAME	GENERIC NAME	DOSAGE	MANUFACTURER
Depo-Estradiol (intramuscular)	Estradiol Cypionate	1mg/ml 5mg/ml	Upjohn
Delestrogen (intramuscular)	Estradiol Valerate	10mg/ml 20mg/ml 40mg/ml	Squibb
Estraval (intramuscular)	Estradiol Valerate	10mg/ml 20mg/ml	Solvay
Premarin (intramuscular and intravenous)	Conjugated Estrogens	25mg/vial	Wyeth-Ayerst
Estrapel (investigational use only in U.S.)	Estradiol Pellet	25mg pellet	Bartor, Progynon
Estraderm	Transdermal	0.05mg patch	Ciba-Geigy
Skin Patch	17-beta Estradiol	0.1 mg patch (release rate per day)	

knowledge. Within ten days of taking the new prescription, the menopausal symptoms began to recur. Switching back to the brand name alleviated the problem.

VARIOUS WAYS IN WHICH ESTROGEN IS ADMINISTERED

How do I know if I am getting the appropriate amount of estrogen to prevent all the menopausal symptoms?

Hot flashes, night sweats, and anxiety symptoms should be relieved. A vaginal estrogen smear can determine the effect of estrogen on the vagina. Estrogen and FSH blood levels can be monitored. Cholesterol profiles can be followed. Periodic bone density measurements can monitor bone loss if that is a concern.

What are the different ways in which estrogen can be administered?

Estrogen can be given orally in the form of a pill, by intramuscular or intravenous injections, by vaginal application with creams or suppositories, by pellets that are implanted beneath the skin in the subcutaneous fat where the hormone is absorbed slowly over several months and by a transdermal skin patch that slowly releases a steady dosage of estrogen over a period of three to four days.

What are the advantages of oral estrogen?

Oral estrogen is the most commonly used, and easiest to administer. In most instances, it is absorbed in a predictable manner. After estrogen is taken orally, it is absorbed by the intestines where it goes into the hepatic (liver) circulation prior to entering the general circulation. Most forms of oral estrogen become metabolized to *estrone* by the liver. It is in this form that estrogen has its effect on the tissues in the body. In going through the liver, estrogen stimulates several of the proteins made in that organ which have both a positive and negative effect on certain bodily functions. The increase in the HDL-cholesterol level is the most positive effect of the first pass through the liver.

What are the disadvantages of the oral estrogen?

Some women do not absorb estrogens well through their intestinal tract. One study showed that as many as 25% of women on estrogen pills do not absorb enough of the hormone to improve their symptoms. If you are taking estrogen and are not helped with your menopausal symptoms, it is possible that the medication is not being absorbed into your general circulation. You may need a higher dosage of estrogen than is usually recommended, or you may have to switch to either an injectable or skin patch method of administration.

Another disadvantage of the oral forms of estrogen is its effect on the liver proteins which may interfere with clotting factors and blood pressure, although this is uncommon in postmenopausal estrogen therapy. Oral estrogen may also cause a slightly higher incidence of gallbladder disease. A non-oral route may be preferable in someone with previous liver disease, blood pressure elevations or thrombophlebitis.

What estrogens are available by injection?

The injectable forms of estrogen include: *estradiol benzoate, polyestradiol phosphate* (Estradurin), *conjugated equine estrogen* (Intravenous Premarin), *estradiol valerate* (Delestrogen, Estate, Gynogen, Menaval), and *estradiol cypionate* (Depo-Estradiol, E-Ionate, E-Cypionate).

What are the advantages and disadvantages of injectable estrogens?

Estrogen injections were more commonly used in the past than at present. Administration of estrogen by a shot does avoid the first pass through the liver, and thus smaller amounts can be given than with oral administration. The drawbacks of injectable administration include the discomfort of the needle, the need to go for injection every three to four weeks, and an initial peak level of estrogen followed by a variable disappearance rate. Once the shot is given, there is no way to stop the medication if a woman has undesirable side effects. It takes three to four weeks before her side effects subside; if she were using estrogen in an oral or skin patch form, it would take only a few days.

The injectable route is often used immediately after surgery (when the body may not tolerate oral medications for several days) if the ovaries are removed, to prevent postoperative hot flashes. The Estraderm skin patch can also be used during the immediate postoperative period. An additional disadvantage of injectable estrogen is suggested by recent evidence that changing levels of estrogen may be responsible for headaches that some women on hormones experience. These women are best treated with a method of estrogen replacement that supplies a steady dose of estrogen, for instance the patch or smaller doses of estrogen pills two or three times per day.

What estrogens are available by the vaginal route?

The vaginal forms of estrogen include: *conjugated equine estrogen* (Premarin), *estropipate* (Ogen), *dinestrol* (DV cream Estragard) and *estradiol* cream (Estrace), and *diethylstibestrol* (generic).

When would vaginal application of estrogen be indicated?

Estrogen is given in cream form usually to counteract vaginal atrophy and dryness. Because the absorption of the

TABLE 3		
ESTROGEN VAGINAL CREAMS		
BRAND NAME	GENERIC NAME	MANUFACTURER
Estrace Vaginal Cream	17beta-estradiol	Mead Johnson
Estragard Cream	Dienestrol	Solvay
Ogen Vaginal Cream	Estropipate	Abbott
Ortho Dienestrol Cream	Dienestrol	Ortho
Premarin Vaginal Cream	Conjugated estrogens	Wyeth-Ayerst
Diethylstilbestrol Suppositories	Diethylstilbestrol	Lilly

cream is unpredictable, with some women absorbing a much higher percentage than others, the vaginal route of administration is not advised for routine estrogen replacement. If you prefer to avoid standard estrogen replacement therapy and have a problem with vaginal atrophy and dryness, small amounts of cream used once or twice a week may be enough to make you more comfortable. If you are using even occasional estrogen vaginal cream, you should be monitored as if you were on replacement therapy, as the vaginal cream, even in small amounts, may stimulate the endometrial lining like other forms of estrogen.

What are the advantages and disadvantages of vaginal estrogen?

Estrogen applied into the vagina by cream or suppository bypasses the liver circulation on the first pass through. It does get absorbed into the general circulation but at an unpredictable rate. Vaginal estrogen has its greatest effect on the vaginal mucosa and is frequently used to treat vaginal atrophy when systemic estrogen is not required. It can also be used as a supplement if vaginal dryness persists while a woman is taking other forms of estrogen.

What is the estrogen skin patch?

The skin patch, called Estraderm, contains *17-B Estradiol,* a natural form of estrogen. This is a relatively new way of taking estrogen. A patch dispensing the required dosage of estrogen is applied to the skin twice a week. Estrogen is released slowly, in a constant dosage, in much the same way that the ovaries release it naturally. In the future we will probably see more hormone preparations in patch form. Combination estrogen and progesterone patches would be ideal for total hormonal replacement.

What are the advantages and disadvantages of the skin patch?

The patch has been effective in controlling hot flashes and for preventing osteoporosis and other menopausal symptoms. It also avoids the first pass through the liver and gives a small, constant dosage of estrogen, which may be better than an injection, in which a large amount disappears at an unpredictable rate. By using the skin patch, a woman with liver disease, high blood pressure, gallbladder disease or thrombophlebitis may still be able to take estrogen without the negative consequences of stimulating the liver proteins.

The disadvantage of the patch is that it does cause skin irritation in a small percentage of women, although there is less chance of irritation if the patch is worn in the buttocks area. Also, by avoiding the first pass through the liver, the patch does not improve the cholesterol to the same degree as the oral route does. The first pass through the liver has the most effect on stimulating the HDL-cholesterol (the good cholesterol).

What are estrogen pellets?

A capsule or pellet of estrogen can be implanted beneath the skin to give a constant low dosage of estrogen. The pellets do relieve hot flashes and do not affect the liver proteins. They also have been shown to prevent calcium loss and osteoporosis. The implants have a variable life span from six to twelve months and can be difficult to remove. It also may be difficult to determine when they need to be replaced. The estrogen pellets are not commonly used at this time, as the FDA has not yet approved them for use in the U.S.

PROGESTINS

What is a progestin?

The term progestin refers to the general class of medications related to progesterone, the hormone normally produced by the corpus luteum of the ovary during a normal menstrual cycle. There are two classes of progestins: those derived from the natural hormone progesterone and those from the hormone testosterone. The progestational medications initially prescribed were derivatives of the male hormone testosterone and *19-nortestosterone*. In addition to their progestational actions, these compounds also had varying degrees of androgenic activity.

What does androgenic mean?

Androgenic refers to a substance which has masculinizing or male-like characteristics. It usually refers to symptoms produced by the male hormone, testosterone. These include: an increase in body mass and weight, acne formation, oily skin, deepening of the voice, and hair growth. The progestational agents derived from testosterone and the 19-nortestosterone compounds are more likely to cause the androgenic side effects than the progestins derived from the natural hormone, progesterone.

Which of the progestins are derived from testosterone and 19-nortestosterone?

Those derived from testosterone and its derivatives include: *dimethisterone, ethynodiol diacetate, norethindrone* (Norlutin, Micronor, Nor-Q.D.), *norethynodrel, norethine-drone acetate* (Norlutate, Aygestin), *norgestrel* (Ovrette), and *l-norgestrel.*

What has been the principal use of the progestational testosterone derivatives?

The progestins derived from the testosterone compounds have been used in oral contraceptives. Recent studies have revealed, however, that small doses of norethindrone (0.7 mg-1.0mg) have been used in postmenopausal women with few side effects. Two of the above preparations (Micronor and Ovrette) are marketed as the progesterone-only birth control pill (often called the mini-pill for women who cannot take estrogen). Levonorgestrel is the hormone in the birth control implant Norplant.

Which progestins are derived from the natural hormone progesterone?

The progestins derived from the natural hormone progesterone include *medroxyprogesterone acetate* (Provera, Amen, Cycrin, Curretabs), *megesterol acetate* (Megace) and *17-a hydoxyprogesterone caproate* (Delalutin). A class of more potent progestins has recently been developed by placing a halogen molecule on the progesterone chemical. These include the preparations *chlormadinone acetate* and *cyproterone acetate.*

How have the natural progestational derivatives been used?

The hormones derived from the natural hormone progesterone have been used for postmenopausal therapy and to

TABLE 4			
PROGESTOGENS			
BRAND NAME	GENERIC NAME	DOSAGE IN MG	MANUFACTURER
Amen	Medroxyprogesterone Acetate	10	Carnick
Curretabs	Medroxyprogesterone Acetate	10	Solvay
Cycrin	Medroxyprogesterone Acetate	10	Wyeth-Ayerst
Provera	Medroxyprogesterone Acetate	2.5, 5, 10	Upjohn
Aygestin	Norethindrone Acetate	5	Wyeth-Ayerst
Norlutate	Norethindrone Acetate	5	Parke-Davis
Norlutin	Norethindrone	5	Parke-Davis
Micronor	Norethindrone	0.35	Ortho
Nor-Q.D.	Norethindrone	0.35	Syntex
Megace	Megesterol Acetate	20, 40	Bristol-Myers
Ovrette	Norgestrel	0.075	Wyeth-Ayerst

treat dysfunctional uterine bleeding during the menstrual years. Most physicians prefer to use medroxyprogesterone acetate (Provera, Amen, Cycrin, Curretabs) in the treatment of postmenopausal women because of the low incidence of side effects.

Why did the use of progestins become popular in estrogen therapy?

The addition of a progestin to estrogen replacement therapy actually reduces the incidence of endometrial hyperplasia and endometrial cancer. For this reason, if you still have your uterus and are on estrogen replacement therapy, you should also take a progestational drug. Most physicians advise women who do not have their uterus to take only estrogen, to avoid the possible negative effect of progestin on the cardiovascular system.

What are the side effects and disadvantages to giving the progestin?

Adding progestin to estrogen, and taking the medication cyclically, will usually cause a return of menstrual periods. Some women are very sensitive to the possible side effects of progestins, which include anxiety, nervousness, moodiness, depression, abdominal bloating, and headaches. In these cases, lowering the dose of the progestin or taking it every two or three months instead of monthly may help lessen the side effects. If this is still not acceptable, taking estrogen alone is an option, as long as a yearly endometrial biopsy or ultrasound exam is performed, to measure the thickness of the uterine lining.

Do the progestins affect lipid metabolism?

The different types of progestins appear to cause dissimilar psychological and metabolic effects. The progestins in general appear to have the opposite effect on cholesterol than estrogen—they lower the HDL-cholesterol level and raise the LDL-cholesterol level, both negative outcomes. Some of the progestins may cancel the positive effect that estrogen has on your cholesterol. The effects of the progestins appear to be related to the dosage, however, so the minimum effective dosage should be prescribed.

Is one progestin more beneficial than another?

Medroxyprogesterone acetate (Provera, Amen, Cycrin, Curretabs) appears to have minimal effect on the cholesterol; therefore, it has been designated by a number of physicians as the drug of choice to be used in postmenopausal therapy. To be totally fair to the other progestational agents, some of the studies relating cholesterol changes to dosage used much higher doses than necessary. Several new progestational agents are still being investigated or awaiting FDA approval for use in both oral contraceptives and postmenopausal hormone therapy. These include micronized progesterone, norgestimate, gestodene, and desogestrel. All of these have been found to have little effect on lipid metabolism and may replace the presently used progestins in the near future.

How long must the progestin be taken to prevent endometrial hyperplasia?

The reduction of hyperplasia and cancer is directly related to the number of days the progestin is taken. The incidence of endometrial hyperplasia, felt to be a precursor to endometrial cancer, was shown to be 18%–32% with estrogen therapy alone. This was reduced to 3%–4% when a progestin was used for seven days and to 2% when a ten-day course was prescribed. A more recent study showed that taking the progestin for 12 to 13 days each month *totally eliminated* the incidence of hyperplasia. Although the most popular regimen has been a 10-day course of therapy, with this recent evidence, it may be best to take the progestin for 12 to 13 days each month. This more closely resembles the progestational phase of the normal menstrual cycle (14 days).

Are there ways to take the progestins other than orally?

Although progesterone preparations can be given by injection, vaginally, or rectally, the only way to cycle women during the menopause with progestins is to prescribe a pill orally. It would be ideal if a progestin could be delivered by a skin patch to avoid the first pass through the liver, as the most negative effect of this medication is its impact on the liver proteins and cholesterol. This may be possible in the near future.

Are progestins beneficial without estrogen for menopausal symptoms?

If you are experiencing bothersome hot flashes and cannot take estrogen, a progestin medication will usually help this condition and can even improve calcium metabolism to prevent osteoporosis. Progestins will not, however, improve vaginal dryness or bladder symptoms related to the menopause and may have a negative effect on the cardiovascular system without the benefit of estrogen.

Who usually takes progestins alone for menopausal symptoms?

The use of progestin therapy alone may be beneficial if you have had cancer of the breast or endometrium and are not a candidate for estrogen therapy. If you are having severe side effects such as breast tenderness, severe fibrocystic breast disease, continual breakthrough bleeding, or nausea from even low-dose estrogen replacement therapy, you may also benefit from progestin therapy.

ANDROGEN USE IN MENOPAUSE

When is testosterone indicated in the menopause?

The use of testosterone is gaining in popularity during the menopausal period. The ovaries in a normal menstruating woman produce a small, but significant, amount of the male hormone testosterone. At the time of a natural menopause and especially after a surgical menopause, the levels of testosterone fall off significantly (much like estrogen levels). When this small amount of testosterone is replaced postmenopausally, women enjoy a stronger sex drive and more energy. Although testosterone during the menopause has been prescribed chiefly to improve a woman's sex drive, some researchers have used the combination estrogen-testosterone preparations routinely in *all women*. They claim that their patients using the combination feel better and have more energy in addition to an increased sex drive.

Can testosterone replace the use of progestin?

Although some progestins have some androgenic effects, the use of testosterone *does not* replace the use of progestin to minimize endometrial hyperplasia of the uterine lining. If a woman has her uterus, she still needs to take a progestin whether she is on estrogen alone or an estrogen-testosterone combination. If she has had a hysterectomy, she should not need the progestin.

What combination preparations are available?

Although testosterone can be prescribed separately, it is more convenient and less expensive to take a combination estrogen-testosterone preparation. There are presently two combination oral preparations available—*Estratest* and *Premarin* with *methyltestosterone*. The dosages of testosterone in the Premarin preparations are 5mg and 10mg combined with 0.625mg and 1.25mg of estrogen respectively. This may be too much testosterone for many woman. Excess testosterone causes some unpleasant side effects, such as weight gain, acne, and hair growth. The dosage in *Estratest* is 1.25mg of estrogen combined with 2.5mg of testosterone and the dosage in *Estratest HS* is 0.625mg of estrogen combined with 1.25mg of testosterone. The latter appears to be better tolerated by many women while achieving the desired effect. An injectable form of the combination is also available (*Depo-testadiol*). If indeed these combinations gain in popularity, we will see

TABLE 5			
ESTROGEN/ANDROGEN COMBINATIONS			
BRAND NAME	ESTROGEN + ANDROGEN	DOSAGE IN MG	MANUFACTURER
Estratest	esterified estrogens + methyl testosterone	1.25 0.625 + + 2.5 1.25	Solvay
Premarin with Methyl Testosterone	conjugated estrogens + methyl testosterone	0.625 1.25 + + 5.0 10	Wyeth-Ayerst
Depo-Testadiol Injectable	estradiol cypionate + testosterone cypionate	2mg + 50mg	Upjohn

more variations available. (See Table 5 for a list of combination estrogen-androgen preparations.)

Are there side effects from testosterone?

The side effects of testosterone include weight gain, acne, hair growth, deepening of the voice, and a negative influence on cholesterol and lipid metabolism. If a person takes enough testosterone, all of the above will result. The low doses of testosterone used in postmenopausal hormone therapy, however, are well tolerated by most women.

REGIMENS OF HORMONAL THERAPY

What is hormonal replacement therapy?

When estrogen is prescribed in the postmenopausal period, it is often referred to as *estrogen replacement therapy* or ERT.

If a combination of estrogen and progesterone is prescribed, it is often referred to as *hormonal replacement therapy* or HRT. The two most common ways to take estrogen and progesterone during menopause are through cyclic and continuous therapy.

What is cyclic therapy?

Cyclic hormonal replacement therapy involves taking estrogen for a certain number of days during the month, followed by 10 to 13 days of a progestin. Here is how it usually works: you take the estrogen for the first 25 calendar days each month accompanied by the progestin from day 13 through day 25. Or to put it another way, you take estrogen alone from the 1st through the 12th day each month. Then, from the 13th to the 25th day, you take estrogen plus the progestin. Your doctor gives you no medication from the 26th day to the end of the month. This will provide 13 days of the progestin each month, which has been shown to help prevent endometrial hyperplasia.

Are there other ways to take cyclic therapy?

Although the regimen described above appears the most popular method of cyclic hormonal therapy, others are available. Some women do not tolerate stopping their estrogen for 5 to 6 days every month because bothersome headaches or hot flashes result. There is no reason that estrogen has to be stopped, as long as the progestin is taken for 10 to 13 days. Therefore, an alternative to the 25-day regimen is to take estrogen *daily* without skipping any days and to pick any 10 to 13 days to take the progestin (usually the first 10 to 13 days of the month). An added benefit of this regimen is that you may delay taking the progestin for a week or so if, for instance, you want to avoid your period while on a trip.

Will I get menstrual bleeding if I follow the cyclic regimen?

About 75% of women experience bleeding after they finish the progestin when on cyclic therapy. The closer you are to menopause, the greater the chance of bleeding. Bleeding does tend to get lighter, however, as the years go by. Bleeding that does not correlate with the progestin phase of your cycle should be investigated with an endometrial biopsy.

What are the standard doses of hormones?

The lowest doses of estrogen that have been shown to treat the majority of menopausal symptoms and prevent osteoporosis are 0.625mg of Premarin or Ogen, 1mg of Estrace, and the 0.05mg Estraderm patch. In any one individual, however, lower or higher doses of these estrogens may be satisfactory, or necessary to control symptoms. The standard dose of medroxyprogesterone acetate (Provera, Cycrin, Amen, Curretabs) has recently been reduced from 10mg to 5mg or 2.5mg for 10 to 13 days each month. Some women do not tolerate progestins at all, so taking estrogen may be an alternative only if followed appropriately. (See page 239.)

Is there a way to prevent menstrual bleeding while on estrogen-progestin therapy?

Lowering the doses of estrogen and progestin may help, but too low a dose may not control all of your symptoms. If osteoporosis is a concern at the lower doses of estrogen, serial bone density measurements can be made to check whether bone loss is occurring. If reducing the doses of estrogen and progestin isn't helpful, continuous therapy may be tried.

What is continuous therapy?

This new approach to estrogen-progestin therapy has been gaining in popularity. It involves taking an estrogen plus a very low dose of progestin on a daily basis all month long. If breakthrough bleeding occurs, the progestin is increased slightly until no bleeding occurs, and then it may be lowered back to the normal dose. Some studies have tried the combined estrogen-progestin therapy just during the week and not on weekend days. This combination lowers the total amount of hormone being ingested, yet has prevented bleeding without evidence of side effects. Individual evaluation is very important, as not all women respond in the same way to similar doses of the same hormones. Adjustments may have to be made that apply best to you.

What is the goal of continuous therapy?

The goal of continuous therapy is to eliminate menstrual bleeding which is the biggest complaint of postmenopausal women on estrogen therapy. The continuous regimen does protect the uterine lining from endometrial hyperplasia and cancer as proven by endometrial biopsies. The dose of progestin necessary to accomplish this is usually lower than that taken in cyclic therapy. Instead of 10mg of medroxyprogesterone acetate, only 2.5mg to 5mg is necessary on a daily basis.

What is the effect of continuous therapy on the cholesterol and lipids?

Since it is the progestin that has the negative effect on lipid metabolism, one would postulate that continuous therapy may increase the LDL-cholesterol level or decrease the HDL-cholesterol level (both negative effects). Using progestins that have little effect on lipids (such medroxyprogesterone acetate) and lowering the dose to the 2.5mg range has revealed no change in the LDL-cholesterol/HDL-cholesterol ratio. The newer progestational drugs, norgestimate and gestodene, have even less affect on lipid metabolism.

Does continuous therapy prevent endometrial hyperplasia?

Studies have shown that, if the right combination of estogen and progestin is used, this regimen will prevent endometrial hyperplasia. The continuous method of taking estrogen and progesterone may be the ideal way of taking hormones during menopause because it avoids the most common complaint of postmenopausal women on hormones—that of continual menstrual periods. It is not necessary to have a period to protect the uterine lining from hyperplasia.

Are there any disadvantages to continuous therapy?

As in other methods of estrogen and progesterone replacement, breakthrough bleeding continues to be the biggest problem. It may take up to six months of nuisance spotting before the uterine lining becomes atrophic enough to discontinue bleeding. If bleeding persists, you may need an endometrial biopsy to ensure the bleeding has no other cause.

Do some women do better than others on continuous therapy?

Women who are several years beyond menopause and whose ovaries have completely stopped producing estrogen generally do better on continuous therapy. Perimenopausal women have more problems with irregular bleeding because, in addition to the hormones they are taking, their own ovaries are still intermittently producing estrogen.

SEEKING TREATMENT

What type of doctor should I see for my menopausal symptoms?

There are many different types of physicians who can manage your care. Although gynecologists have been considered specialists in the health care of women, many other physicians should be able to help you with your symptoms. Much will depend on your physician's experience and interest in managing your problems. Many primary care physicians, such as family doctors and internal medicine specialists (general internists, endocrinologists, and geriatric specialists) may be experienced in managing the menopausal syndrome. A gynecologist may have the most overall experience in managing menopausal symptoms especially related to bleeding abnormalities and hormonal therapy during the menopausal years. At times, your treatment may involve coordinated care from several different specialists, such as a gynecologist, internist, endocrinologist, psychologist, or psychiatrist. Don't be afraid to discuss your symptoms with your doctor. If you aren't satisfied, seek another opinion.

What type of exam should I have if I am going to start and continue on hormonal replacement therapy?

A general physical exam including your blood pressure, urinalysis, pelvic, pap smear, and breast exam should be performed at least yearly. Some physicians may want to see you more often when hormonal therapy is first started. Mammograms should be performed according to the American Cancer Society's guidelines with a yearly mammogram after 50, especially if you are on hormonal therapy. A cholesterol screening with a breakdown of the HDL and LDL cholesterol levels, if the total cholesterol is elevated, should also be performed. If the results of these are abnormal, appropriate diet and management suggestions should be followed. A complete general physical exam including an electrocardiogram, chest X-ray and proctologic exam should also be performed at appropriate intervals. Not all physicians agree upon the frequency of some of these studies. If you are at risk for osteoporosis, a bone densiometer study should be performed.

What can I do to help ease my transition into menopause?

You can do many things for yourself. Avoid smoking and excessive alcohol and caffeine. A diet low in cholesterol and fats, an adequate intake of calcium and an appropriate exercise program to stimulate your bones and cardiovascular system should all help maximize your enjoyment during the postmenopausal years. Serious consideration should be given to hormone replacement therapy; weigh its advantages and disadvantages in your particular case. If you are having bothersome symptoms, or are at risk for osteoporosis or cardiovascular disease, hormonal therapy can make a difference between an enjoyable life and just existing.

Glossary

Abortion—The premature loss of a pregnancy.

Absorptiometry—A technique utilizing low-energy radioisotopes to measure the density of bone. This process is used to measure the degree of osteoporosis present in bone.

Adenoma—A benign growth or tumor arising from an epithelial surface such as an adematous polyp.

Adenocarcinoma—A cancerous growth arising from an adenoma such as an adenocarcinoma of the endometrium (uterine lining).

Adenomyosis—A condition in which the uterine lining tissue (endometrium) grows into the uterine muscle wall, possibly causing heavy menstrual periods; often referred to as internal endometriosis.

Adrenal glands—These small glands are situated above each kidney and are responsible for controlling sugar and salt metabolism. They also secrete androgenic (male-like) hormones which the body fat converts to estrogen.

Adrenocorticotropic hormone (ACTH)—Hormone produced by the pituitary gland that regulates the hormonal production of the adrenal gland.

Amenorrhea—Absence or cessation of a woman's period.

Amenorrhea galactorrhea—A milky secretion from the breasts (galactorrhea) that sometimes occurs with the cessation of menstrual periods. This may be caused by an elevated level of the hormone prolactin from a pituitary gland tumor.

Androgenic—A substance or hormone that produces male or masculine characteristics.

Androgens—The male sex hormones or their derivatives that produce masculine characteristics.

Andropause—The "male menopause" that occurs in men in their 60s and is characterized by a decrease in the production of male hormones (androgens), decreased sex drive, hot flashes, restlessness, and sleepless nights.

Anesthesia—The loss of feeling or sensation. General anesthesia refers to total loss of consciousness or "being put to sleep." Local or regional anesthesia refers to the anesthetizing of a specific region or area of the body such as a spinal anesthetic. During local anesthesia, the patient is usually conscious and alert.

Angina pectoris—Chest pain caused by insufficient oxygen reaching the heart muscle; often a precursor to a heart attack.

Anovulation—The suspension or cessation of ovulation.

Atherosclerosis—A disease of the arteries in which fatty plaques develop on their interior walls, with eventual obstruction of blood flow; also known as "hardening of the arteries."

Atrophic vaginitis—An inflammation of the vagina caused by a thinning of the vaginal wall due to a lack of estrogen; also called senile and postmenopausal vaginitis.

Axillary lymph nodes—The lymph nodes under the arm which are often removed during a breast biopsy or breast cancer operation to determine if the cancer has spread.

Bellergal—A medication used to treat hot flashes in women who are not candidates for estrogen therapy.

Biopsy—The removal and examination of tissue from the body to make a diagnosis.

Breast—The mammary gland in mammals.

Calcitonin—A hormone produced by the thyroid gland that is important in bone metabolism.

Calcium—A mineral that is crucial to the body for the prevention of osteoporosis.

Cancer—An abnormal growth of cells which destroy the body's vital organs and ultimately can cause death.

Cardiovascular diseases—Any disease that affects the circulation of blood and oxygen through the heart and blood vessels.

Cauterization—The burning or application of a caustic substance to destroy tissue. It is commonly used on the cervix to treat chronic cervicitis or on the Fallopian tubes for sterilization.

Cervical canal polyps—Benign growths that begin in the endocervical canal and may protrude through the cervix causing abnormal bleeding.

Cervical conization—Surgical procedure in which a cone-shaped piece of tissue is removed from the center of the cervix. It is usually performed when a Pap smear reveals abnormal cells present in the endocervical canal.

Cervicitis—Inflammation or infection of the cervix that may cause an abnormal discharge.

Cervix—The neck of the uterus that protrudes into the vagina. The cells used for a Pap smear are taken from this part of the uterus.

Chocolate cyst—An ovarian cyst filled with old, dried blood resembling chocolate. It usually results from endometriosis of the ovaries and is also called an endometrioma.

Cholesterol—A fatty substance needed by the body for normal function. If present in excessive amounts and deposited in the arteries, it leads to atherosclerosis (hardening of the arteries) and heart attacks.

Climacteric—The period of time in a woman's life in which her body undergoes changes from a reproductive to a nonreproductive state, usually between the ages of 40 and 60.

Clitoris—The female counterpart of the penis; like the penis, it is extremely sensitive and becomes erect during sexual stimulation.

Clonidine—A medication used to treat high blood pressure which has also been shown to help hot flashes in women who cannot take estrogen.

Collagen—A major fibrous protein which is the main supportive substance of skin, bone, tendons, cartilage, and connective tissue.

Colles fracture—A fracture of the wrist, common in women who develop osteoporosis.

Colposcopy—A medical procedure in which a telescope-like instrument is used to look at the cervix and vagina to locate abnormal cells found on a Pap smear.

Conception—The fertilization of the egg by the sperm, which results in pregnancy. To conceive means to become pregnant.

Condom—A sheath placed on a man's erect penis before intercourse to prevent sperm from entering the vagina; a commonly used method of birth control in perimenopausal women.

Conjugated equine estrogens—A mixture of estrogens derived from pregnant mares' urine used in hormonal replacement therapy. It was one of the original estrogens available for estrogen replacement and is used as the standard when compared to other estrogen preparations. Premarin is the most commonly known conjugated estrogen.

Conservative surgery—A term used for endometriosis surgery performed on the uterus, tubes and ovaries to preserve childbearing capability by not removing the pelvic organs.

Contraception—The practice of using a device, drug, or procedure to prevent pregnancy.

Contraceptive—Anything used to prevent pregnancy.

Contraceptive jelly—A jelly that kills sperm; it is used in association with a diaphragm to prevent pregnancy.

Contraceptive sponge—A small sponge that contains a spermicide; when placed in the vagina against the cervix, it acts as a barrier method of birth control.

Coronary arteries—The arteries that supply the heart muscle with oxygen and nutrients.

Coronary heart disease—Another term for diseases of the heart caused by diseases of the coronary arteries.

Coronary insufficiency—A condition that results from insufficient oxygen reaching the heart muscle causing angina pectoris (chest pain).

Corpus luteum—The organ that forms in the ovary after ovulation has occurred. It produces the hormone progesterone which is vital to counteract the estrogen build-up to the uterine lining.

Corpus luteal cyst—A cyst that may form from the corpus luteum; along with a follicular cyst, it is one of the functional cysts of the ovary.

Cryosurgery—Surgical procedure that utilizes freezing to remove abnormal tissue. It is often used to treat abnormal cells or excessive mucus-secreting cells on the cervix.

CT-scan—A diagnostic X-ray procedure that uses computers to project an image on film.

Cyst—A sac that contains a liquid or semi-solid substance. Some cysts, especially on the ovary, are related to normal ovarian function while other cysts can be a sign of an abnormal growth or tumor.

Cystocele—The herniation of the urinary bladder into the anterior part of the vagina.

D & C—Dilatation and curettage.

Danazol—A synthetic androgenic medication that causes a pseudomenopause. It is used to treat endometriosis and some cases of severe fibrocystic breast disease.

Depo-Provera—An injectable, long-acting progesterone used to treat endometriosis, irregular menses and other gynecologic conditions.

Dermis—The deeper part of the skin which contains most of the skin's vital sturctures. Ninety-seven percent of the dermis consists of the protein, collagen.

Diaphragm—A molded rubber cap used with contraceptive jelly to provide a barrier method of contraception.

Diethylstilbestrol (DES)—A synthetic female hormone used during the 1940s and 1950s to treat abnormal bleeding during pregnancy and threatened miscarriages. It subsequently was found to cause abnormalities in the male and female genital tract of the offspring who were exposed in utero.

Dilatation and curettage (D&C)—A surgical procedure in which the cervix is dilated to allow a spoon-shaped instrument (curette) into the uterus to scrape the uterine lining. It is used to treat and diagnose abnormal uterine bleeding and to remove remaining pregnancy tissue after a miscarriage.

Dysfunctional uterine bleeding—Abnormal uterine bleeding (irregular periods) without an apparent cause; usually attributed to an abnormal and irregular hormone production from the ovaries.

Dysmenorrhea—Painful menstrual periods.

Dyspareunia—Painful intercourse.

Dysuria—Painful urination.

Ectopic pregnancy—A pregnancy that implants and grows anywhere other than in the uterine cavity. Most commonly occurs in the Fallopian tube but may occur on the ovary, cervix or abdominal cavity.

Elective abortion—The elective termination of a pregnancy.

Endocrine gland—A gland that secretes hormones that have a specific effect on another organ of the body. The pituitary, thyroid, adrenal, and hypothalmus glands, as well as the ovaries, are all endocrine glands and are part of the reproductive system.

Endometrial aspiration—An aspiration or suction of the uterine lining to obtain tissue for diagnosis and treat abnormal uterine bleeding; often called an "office D & C."

Endometrial biopsy—A biopsy of the endometrium to determine abnormalities within the uterus.

Endometrioma—A growth or cyst in the ovary consisting of endometriosis and dried blood; often referred to as a chocolate cyst of the ovary.

Endometriosis—A condition in which tissue resembling the endometrium occurs outside the uterus, such as on the ovaries, Fallopian tubes, and pelvic ligaments. In the perimenopausal woman, it may cause severe pain with ovarian cysts and may be an indication for a hysterectomy.

Endometrium—The lining of the internal surface of the uterus which is shed when a woman has her menstrual period.

Endoscope—An instrument connected to a fiberoptic light source used to examine the inside of an organ. Examples of endoscopes are: a cystoscope, used to look inside the bladder; a hysteroscope, used to look inside the uterus; and a laparoscope, used to look inside the abdominal and pelvic cavity.

Enterocele—A herniation of the intestines into the top of the vaginal vault.

Entero-hepatic circulation (intestinal-liver circulation)—An oral medication, such as estrogen, is absorbed by the intestinal tract and goes to the liver via the portal vein where it is metabolized prior to entering the general circulation.

Epidermis—The superfical part of the skin which overlies and protects the dermis. It produces keratin which gives the skin its protective covering.

ERT—An abbreviation for estrogen replacement therapy.

Estrogen—A group of female hormones, produced by the ovaries, that are responsible for a woman's female characteristics, such as breast development and menstruation. The lack of estrogen causes menopause and its related symptoms.

Estrogen index—A test used to determine the level of estrogen present in the vagina; also called the maturation index.

Fallopian tubes—The long, slender tubes that extend from the upper lateral angle of the uterus toward the ovaries on each side. The tubes pick up the egg after ovulation. Fertilization normally occurs within them.

Fertilization—The uniting of the sperm with the egg which results in the start of a pregnancy.

Fibrocystic breast disease—A condition of the breast in which an abundance of cystic structures arise from the glands within the breast tissue.

Fibroid tumor—A growth of uterine muscle fibers resulting in a benign tumor. Also called a myoma or leiomyoma. They range in size from as small as a pea to as large as a basketball.

Fibrosarcoma—A cancerous fibroid tumor.

Fimbria—The finger-like projections at the end of the Fallopian tube.

Follicular stimulating hormone (FSH)—A hormone secreted by the pituitary gland that causes an egg within the ovary to mature. It is controlled by the estrogen produced by the egg within the ovary and rises to very high levels when the ovaries no longer produce estrogen. An elevated FSH is one way your doctor can determine if you have reached menopause.

Formication—A rare menopausal symptom in which a woman feels as if insects are crawling all over her skin.

Fracture—A break in a bone.

Frequency—A term used to refer to urinating frequently; often associated with urgency and dysuria as part of the senile urethral syndrome.

Functional ovarian cyst—An ovarian cyst related to the normal function of the ovaries; a corpus luteal or graffian follicular cyst.

Galactorrhea—Excessive or spontaneous flow of milk from the breast. In the non-pregnant state, it may be the sign of a small pituitary gland tumor called a microadenoma.

Gallbladder—A sac located on the under surface of the liver which stores the bile helpful in the digestion of fats.

Gonadotropin releasing hormone (GnRH)—A hormone produced by the hypothalmus that stimulates the pituitary gland to produce FSH and LH.

Graafian follicle—The follicle within the ovary in which the egg is produced and estrogen is made. After ovulation the Graafian follicle becomes a corpus luteum which then produces progesterone.

Gynecologist—A physician who treats conditions and diseases of the female reproductive system.

HDL-cholesterol—The high density lipoprotein cholesterol or the "good cholesterol"; it carries cholesterol away from the tissue for excretion from the body. It is best to have high HDL cholesterol.

Hormone—A chemical substance secreted by an endocrine gland that affects other organs. GnRH, FSH, LH, estrogen, progesterone and testosterone are all hormones related to the female reproductive system in the perimenopausal woman.

Hot flash—A common perimenopausal symptom in which there is a feeling of intense heat, coupled with redness and perspiration over a woman's body.

Hot flush—The hot flash as visualized by another person and is the British term for a hot flash.

HRT— An abbreviation for hormonal replacement therapy; the use of both estrogen and progesterone, and possibly androgen, as hormone replacement therapy in the menopause in contrast to ERT, which stands for estrogen replacement therapy and refers to estrogen alone.

Hyperplasia—An abnormal increase in the number of cells within an organ. If it occurs within the uterine lining it is called endometrial hyperplasia. If the cells become atypical, it may lead to cancer of the uterine lining.

Hypothalmus—An area in the brain which controls the reproductive system in men and women. It produces GnRH which controls the pituitary gland and ovaries and is also the center for temperature control in the body. The instability of the hypothalmus is theorized to cause hot flashes in the menopausal woman.

Hysterectomy—The surgical removal of the uterus.

Hysteroscopy—A procedure used to look directly inside the uterine cavity by using an instrument called a hysteroscope connected to a fiberoptic light source. It is also the instrument a laser beam is directed through to perform a "laser hysterectomy."

Insomnia—The inability to sleep.

Intrauterine device (IUD)—A device inserted into the uterine cavity to prevent pregnancy.

Kegel exercises—Exercises used to strengthen the muscles around the urethra, bladder, and rectum to increase the tone of the muscles to prevent stress incontinence.

Labia majora—The hairy outer folds on each side of the vagina that contain the sebaceous and sweat glands; often called the outer lips of the vulva.

Labia minora—The thin skin folds inside the labia majora; often called the inner lips of the vulva.

Laparoscopy—A surgical procedure in which a fiberoptic endoscope, called a laparoscope, is inserted through the umbilicus (navel) to look directly at the uterus, Fallopian tubes and ovaries. The procedure has many uses—diagnosing pelvic pain, looking for endometriosis, performing female sterilization, and differentiating the origin of a pelvic mass in the ovaries or uterus.

Laser surgery—Surgery utilizing a laser beam to destroy tissue; usually utilized by surgeons through endoscopes, such as a hysteroscope or laparoscope.

LDL-cholesterol—The low density lipoprotein cholesterol; it deposits cholesterol in the walls of the blood vessels in our body. It is best to have low LDL cholesterol.

Leiomyoma—A benign muscle growth of the uterine muscle; also called fibroids or myomas.

Lipids—The fatty substances in our bloodstream consisting of cholesterol and triglycerides.

Lipoproteins—The proteins in the bloodstream which carry the lipids.

Liver—A large gland located in the right upper quadrant of the abdominal cavity responsible for many bodily functions. It manufactures cholesterol and many proteins crucial for the body to function.

Lumpectomy—The surgical removal of a lump or tumor.

Luteal phase defect—A condition in which there is an inadequate production of progesterone by the corpus luteum of the ovary after ovulation. It may result in infertility or early spontaneous miscarriages if a woman is trying to get pregnant, or irregular menstrual bleeding in the perimenopausal woman.

Luteinizing hormone (LH)—A hormone produced by the pituitary gland that triggers ovulation; along with FSH controls the ovulation and estrogen production by the ovaries.

Lymph nodes—A node of tissue which drains the lymph from our system prior to entering the blood.

Mammogram—An X-ray of the breasts utilized in screening for very early breast cancer.

Marshall-Marchetti operation—An operation through an abdominal incision to support the urinary bladder for the treatment of stress incontinence.

Mastectomy—The surgical removal of the breast.

Maturation index—A test utilizing cells from the vaginal wall to determine the amount of estrogen stimulation to the vagina; also called estrogen index.

Medical D & C—The use of progesterone either orally or by injection to cause a withdrawal menstrual period; often used to treat dysfunctional uterine bleeding.

Menarche—A woman's first menstrual period.

Menopause—A woman's last menstrual period.

Menses—The monthly flow of blood from a woman's uterus; the shedding of the uterine lining. Also called menstruation or a menstrual period.

Microcalcifications—Small deposits of calcium which may be a sign of early breast cancer if found on a mammogram.

Mucosa—The mucous membrane or internal lining of an organ.

Myocardial infarction—A heart attack caused by a blockage of one of the coronary arteries or its branches.

Myoma—A benign tumor of the uterine muscle fibers; also called a fibroid tumor or leiomyoma.

Myomectomy—A surgical procedure in which myomas are removed from the uterus, preserving the uterus for future childbearing.

Oligomenorrhea—Infrequent menstrual bleeding due to irregular ovulation.

Oligoovulation—Ovulation which occurs only once every several months.

Oophorectomy—The surgical removal of the ovaries; unilateral oophorectomy is removal of one ovary, bilateral oophorectomy is removal of both ovaries.

Oral contraceptive—The birth control pill.

Orgasm—The peak of sexual excitement or sexual climax.

Osteoblast—The bone cell responsible for laying down new bone in the continual process of bone remodeling.

Osteoclast—The bone cell responsible for absorbing bone in the continual process of bone remodeling.

Osteoporosis—The process in which bone loss exceeds bone production resulting in very thin bones susceptible to fracture.

Ovarian cyst—A sac-like structure in the ovary that causes an enlargement of the ovary. An ovarian cyst may have many causes, some related to the normal function of the ovary (follicular and corpus luteal cysts) and others caused by benign or malignant tumors of the ovary.

Ovarian failure—The time when the ovaries stop producing estrogen, also called menopause. If menopause occurs before the age of 40, it is referred to as premature menopause or premature ovarian failure.

Ovary—The female sexual gland that produces eggs as well as the hormones estrogen and progesterone.

Ovulation—The discharge of a ripe, unfertilized egg from the ovary.

Ovum—The female reproductive cell or egg.

Pap smear—A test in which cells are removed from the cervix and placed on a slide for microscopic examination. The test is used to diagnose cancerous and precancerous conditions of the cervix. Named after the Greek physician, George N. Papanicolaou.

Pathologist—A physician trained in diagnosing cellular structure of disease. A pathologist reads Pap smears and biopsies and examines tissue after it is removed at surgery to determine if it is cancerous.

Pelviscopy—An expanded laparoscopy procedure utilizing multiple secondary incisions to perform pelvic surgery, such as removing ectopic pregnancies or ovaries through small incisions rather than a full abdominal incision.

Perimenopause—The few years prior to the last menstrual period.

Perineorrhaphy—A surgical procedure to tighten the vaginal opening by removing the excess skin around it.

Pessary—An instrument placed within the vagina to support the bladder, vagina, and rectum; utilized in non-surgical candidates with cystocele, rectoceles, and uterine prolapse.

Pituitary gland—A small gland in the brain located between and behind the eyes that secretes hormones to control many other important glands in the body, including the ovaries, thyroid and adrenal glands.

Polyp—A growth arising from the mucus membrane of a body cavity. The most common type of polyp related to the female reproductive system occurs in the uterine cavity and may cause abnormal bleeding.

Postmenopausal—The time after a woman's last menstrual period.

Progestin—A hormone related to the hormone progesterone.

Prolactin—A hormone produced by the pituitary gland which causes a woman to lactate. It can also be produced by small tumors of the pituitary gland and causes amenorrhea (no periods) and a milky secretion from the breast called galactorrhea.

Prostaglandin—A hormone produced by the uterine lining at the time of a menstrual period; responsible for the severe cramps some women experience at the time of their period.

Premature menopause—Menopause which occurs before the age of 40; also called premature ovarian failure.

Progesterone—The hormone produced by the corpus luteum of the ovary after a woman ovulates. The sudden fall in progesterone production brings on a menstrual period. The irregular production of progesterone is one of the principle causes of irregular menstrual bleeding in the perimenopausal woman.

Pseudomenopause—A condition created when danazol is used to treat endometriosis or fibrocystic breast disease. It may cause symptoms similar to menopause—hot flashes, vaginal dryness, and breast atrophy.

Puberty—The onset of sexual development in a child.

Radiologist—A physician who reads X-rays.

Rectocele—A herniation of the rectum through the posterior vaginal wall.

Salpingectomy—The surgical removal of the Fallopian tube. A partial salpingectomy is performed with some types of female sterilization.

Salpingoophorectomy—The surgical removal of the Fallopian tubes and ovaries. If one ovary and tube are removed, the procedure is referred to as a unilateral salpingoophorectomy; if both are removed, it is called a bilateral salpingoophorectomy.

Senile urethral syndrome—The symptoms of urinary frequency, urgency, and painful urination attributed to the thinning of the urethra from a lack of estrogen.

Spinnbarkeit—The elasticity or stretchiness of the cervical mucus which peaks at the time of ovulation in a woman's menstrual cycle.

Sterilization—A permanent form of birth control accomplished by a vasectomy in the male or a tubal ligation in the female.

Stress inconinence—The loss of urine associated with an increase in intraabdominal pressure, such as in coughing, sneezing, or jumping rope.

Stroke—A form of vascular disease caused by a blockage of one of the arteries going to the brain. The symptoms depend on what part of the brain is affected.

Stroma—The supporting tissue around the glands of an organ. The stroma within the ovaries is where testosterone is produced.

Testosterone—The male hormone produced by the testicles in men. Women also have a smaller amount of testosterone produced by the ovaries and, in some cases, its lack may be responsible for a decreased sex drive in postmenopausal women.

Thrombophlebitis—The inflammation or formation of clots within a vein.

Thyroid gland—A large gland located in front of and on each side of the trachea that secretes thyroxin, the thyroid hormone that controls the body's metabolism.

Trigone—The base of the urinary bladder that rests on top of the vaginal wall. It is very sensitive to estrogen.

Tubal sterilization—A permanent method of birth control in the female by tying, ligating, cauterizing or banding the Fallopian tubes.

Turner's Syndrome—A woman with an XO (rather than the normal XX) sex-chromosome pattern characterized by short stature, webbed neck, an increased carrying angle of the elbow, and a lack of sexual development. Turners's mosaicism (a mixture of XX and XO chromosomes) may be responsible for premature menopause in some women.

Ultrasound examination—An examination utilizing sound waves to produce an image on a monitor. Pelvic ultrasound is often used to help delineate abnormal masses within the pelvis and to determine their exact size.

Unopposed estrogen therapy—Estrogen therapy given alone without a progestin.

Urethra—The membranous canal that carries urine from the bladder to the exterior of the body. The female urethra is sensitive to estrogen deficiency at the time of menopause. This may result in a "senile or atrophic urethral syndrome."

Urethritis—An inflammation or infection of the urethra.

Urinary bladder—The membranous sac above the uterus and vagina which stores the urine before it is excreted from the body.

Urogenital sinus—The embryologic origin of the vagina, bladder, and urethra; all of which are sensitive to estrogen.

Uterine polyp—A growth of the uterine lining which may cause abnormal uterine bleeding; also called an endometrial polyp.

Uterine prolapse—A condition in which the uterus, usually situated in the upper part of the vagina, descends into the lower part of the vagina or even outside the vaginal opening.

Uterus—The hollow muscular organ in a woman that is the place in which a baby develops. It consists of the body, the cervix (neck), and the endometrium (uterine lining).

Vagina—The canal in the female extending from the vulva to the cervix which receives the penis during intercourse. It is extremely sensitive to a lack of estrogen at the time of menopause.

Vaginitis—The inflammation or infection of the vagina. If it is caused by a lack of estrogen, it is called atrophic, senile, or postmenopausal vaginitis.

Vasectomy—A surgical prodedure in which the vas deferens in the male is cut for sterilization purposes.

Vulva—A woman's external genital organs including the mons pubis, labia majora, labia minora, and other structures between the labia.

Womb—The lay term for a woman's uterus.

References

American Cancer Society: *Cancer Facts and Figures.* New York American Cancer Society, 1987.

Ariel IM, Cleary JB (ed): *Breast Cancer: Diagnosis and Treatment.* New York, McGraw Hill, 1987.

Bush TL, Barrett-Conner E, Cowan DK et al: Cardiovascular mortality and noncontraceptive use of estrogen in women: results from the Lipids Research Clinics Program Follow-up Study. *Circulation* 1987;75:1102.

Bush TL, Barrett-Conner E: Noncontraceptive estrogen use and cardiovascular disease. *Epi Rev* 1985;7:80-104.

Campbell S, Whitehead M: Oestrogen therapy and the menopausal syndrome. *Clin Obstet Gynaecol* 1977;4:31-47.

Christianson C, Christensen MS, Transbol I et al: Bone mass in post-menopausal women after withdrawal of oestrogen/gestagen replacement therapy. *Lancet* 1981;1:459-461.

Conference on Menopause: April 21-22, 1988; National Institutes of Health, Bethesda, Maryland.

Eisenberg, M: Endometrial laser ablation for menorrhagia: An effective alternative to hysterectomy. *The Female Patient* 1988; Vol.13, No.5:38-49.

Fisher B, Redmond C, Fisher ER, et al: Ten-year results of a randomized clinical trial comparing radical mastectomy and total mastectomy with or without radiation. *N Engl J Med* 1985;312:665.

Gambrell RD: The menopause. *Invest Radiol* 1986;21:369-378.

Gambrell RD: The role of progestogens in estrogen replacement. *Obstet Gynecol Forum* 1988; Vol 2, No.4:3-13.

Goldrath MH, Fuller TA: Laser photovaporization of endometrium for the treatment of menorrhagia. *Am J Obstet Gynecol* 1981;140:14-19.

Hammond CB, Jelovsek FR, Lee KL et al: Effects of long-term estrogen replacement therapy. I. Metabolic effects. *Am J Obstet Gynecol* 1979; 133:525-547.

Hammond CB, Jelovsek FR, Lee KL et al: Effects of long-term estrogen replacement therapy. II. Neoplasia. *Am J Obstet Gynecol* 1979; 133:537-547.

Hammond CB, Maxson WS: Current status of estrogen therapy for the menopause. *Fertil Steril* 1982;37:5-25.

Henderson BE, Ross RK, Lobo RA et al: Re-evaluating the role of progestogen therapy after the menopause. *Fertil Steril* 1988;49 (supp):9s-13s.

Henderson BE, Ross RK, Paganini-Hill A: Estrogen use and cardiovascular disease. *J Reprod Med* 1985;30:814-820.

Jensen GF, Christiansen C, Transbol I: Treatment of postmenopausal osteoporosis. A controlled therapeutic trial comparing oestrogen/gestagen, 1,25-dihydroxy-vitamin D and calcium. *Clin Endocrinol* 1982; 16:515-524.

Jensen J, Riis BJ, Strom V et al: Long-term effects of percutaneous estrogens and oral progesterone on serum lipoproteins in postmenopausal women. *Am J Obstet Gynecol* 1987; 156:66-71.

Kannel WB, Castelli WP, Gordon T: Cholesterol in the prediction of atherosclerotic disease. New perspectives based on the Framingham study. *Ann Intern Med* 1979;90:85-91.

Kaufman DW, Miller DR, Rosenberg L et al: Noncontraceptive estrogen use and the risk of breast cancer. *JAMA* 1984;252:63-67.

Kopans DB, Meyer JE, Sadowsky N: Breast Imaging. *N Eng J Med* 1984; 310:960-967.

Laufer LR, DeFazio JL, Lu JK, et al: Estrogen replacement therapy by transdermal estradiol administration. *Am J Obstet Gynecol* 1985; 146:533-540.

Limited surgery and radiotherapy for early breast cancer (special report). *N Engl J Med* 1985; 313:1365.

Lindsay R, Hart DM, Clark DM: The minimum effective dose of estrogen for prevention of postmenopausal bone loss. *Obstet Gynecol* 1984; 63:759-763.

Lindsay R, Hart DM, Forrest C et al: Prevention of spinal osteoporosis in oophorectomized women. *Lancet* 1980; 2:1151-1154.

Lomano JM: Photocoagulation of the endometrium with laser for the treatment of menorrhagia. *J Reprod Med* 1986;31:148-150.

Lynch HT, Pennisi VR, Lynch JF: Heredity in breast cancer. In:Ariel IM(ed): *Breast Cancer, Diagnosis and Treatment* New York:McGraw-Hill Co., Chapter 4, 1987.

Mashchak CA, Lobo R: Estrogen replacement therapy and hypertension. *J Reprod Med* 1985;30(supp):805-810.

McDonald DC, Annegers JF, O'Fallon WM et al: Association of exogenous estrogen and endometrial carcinoma: Case-control and incidence study. *AM J Obstet Gynecol* 1977; 127:572-580.

Mishell DR: Estrogen replacement therapy. Measuring benefit vs. cardiovascular risk. *J Reprod Med* 1985;30 (suppl):795-796.

Mishell DR (ed):*Menopause: Physiology and Pharmocology*. Chicago: Year Book Medical Publishers, 1987.

Nachtigall LE, Nachtigall RH, Nachtigall RD et al: Estrogen replacement therapy I: A 10-year prospective study in the relationship to osteoporosis. *Obstet Gynecol* 1979; 53:277-281.

Nachtigall LE, Nachtigall RH, Nachtigall RD et al: Estrogen replacement therapy II: A prospective study in the relationship to carcinoma and cardiovascular and metabolic problems. *Obstet Gynecol* 1979; 54:74-79.

Nambudiri DE, Shamoian CA, Jain HC: Sexuality after menopause. *The Female Patient* 1987; 12:20-26.

Padwick ML, Endacott J, Whitehead MI: Efficacy, acceptability, and metabolic effects of transdermal estradiol in the management of postmenopausal women. *Am J Obstet Gynecol* 1985; 152:1085-1091.

Place VA, Powers M, Darley PE et al: A double-blind comparative study of Estraderm and Premarin in the amelioration of postmenopausal symptoms. *Am J Obstet Gynecol* 1985; 152:1092-1106.

Prough SG, Aksel S, Wiebe RH, et al: Continuous estrogen/progestin therapy in menopause. *Am J Obstet Gynecol* 1987; 157:1449.

Queenan, JT (ed): Special issue, The woman over 50. *Contemporary Ob/Gyn* April 15, 1988; 31.

Shapiro S, Kelly JP, Rosenberg L et al: Risk of localized and widespread endometrial cancer in relation to recent and discontinued use of conjugated estrogens. *New Engl J Med* 1985;313:969-972.

Sherwin BB, Gelfand, MD: The role of androgen in the maintenance of sexual functioning in oophorectomized women. *Psycho Med* 1987;49:397-409.

Sherwin BB, Gelfand MD, Schucher R: Postmenopausal estrogen and androgen replacement and lipoprotein lipid concentrations. *Am J Ob Gyn* 1987;4:414-419.

Smith DC, Prentice R, Thompson DJ et al: Association of exogenous estrogen and endometrial carcinoma. *N Engl J Med* 1975;293:1164-1167.

Speroff L: Androgens in the menopause (symposium proceedings). March 26, 1988; Atlanta, Georgia.

Speroff L: Update on estrogen-progestin replacement therapy. *Postgrad Obstet Gynecol* 1986;6:1-6.

Stampfer MJ, Willett WC, Colditz GA et al: A prospective study of postmenopausal estrogen therapy and coronary heart disease. *N Engl J Med* 1985;313:1044-1049.

Sullivan JM, Zwaag RV, Lemp GF et al: Postmenopausal estrogen use and coronary atherosclerosis. *Ann Int Med* 1988; 108:358-363.

Teran A, Greenblatt RB: Estrogen replacement for the menopause: What to do about it? *Obstet Gynec Forum* 1987; Vol 1, No.6:5-11.

Varma TR: Effect of long-term therapy with estrogen and progesterone on the endometrium of postmenopausal women. *Acta Obstet Gynecol Scand* 1985;64:41-46.

Weiss JS, Ellis CN, Headington JT, Voorhees JJ et al: Topical tretinoin improves photoaged skin. *JAMA* 1988; 259:527-532.

Walsh B, Schiff I: Progestin therapy after the menopause: When is it necessary? *Obstet Gyn Forum* 1988; Vol 2, No.4:2-13.

Wingo PA, Layde PM, Lee NC et al: The risk of breast cancer in post-menopausal women who have used estrogen replacement therapy. *JAMA* 1987;257:209-215.

Ziel HK, Finkle WD: Increased risk of endometrial carcinoma among users of conjugated estrogens. *N Engl J Med* 1975;293:1167-1170.

Index

Books for a healthier and happier life

Arthritis: Don't Learn to Live With It by Carlton Fredericks, Ph.D.
A safe, nutritional approach to treating a crippling disease.

Complete Guide to Symptoms, Illness & Surgery for People Over 50
by H. Winter Griffith, M.D.
The most comprehensive medical reference available for older Americans.

Fitness Walking for Women by Anne Kashiwa and James Rippe, M.D.
A walking program tailored specifically to women's needs and concerns.

Hysterectomy: Making a Choice by Martin D. Greenberg, M.D., P.C.
The first book to deal with alternatives to hysterectomy, written by a leading gynecologist.

Stay Cool Through Menopause by Melvin Frisch, M.D.
A doctor gives up-to-date, clear, detailed answers to the most frequently asked questions about menopause.

These books are available at your bookstore or wherever books are sold, or, for your convenience, we'll send them directly to you. Just call 1-800-631-8571 (press 1 for inquiries and orders) or fill out the coupon below and send it to:

The Putnam Publishing Group
390 Murray Hill Parkway, Dept. B
East Rutherford, NJ 07073

		Price	
		U.S.	Canada
_____ Arthritis: Don't Learn to Live With It	399-51133-4	$ 8.95	$11.75
_____ Complete Guide to Symptoms, Illness & Surgery for People Over 50	399-51749-9	18.95	24.95
_____ Fitness Walking for Women	399-51407-4	9.95	12.95
_____ Hysterectomy: Making a Choice	399-51806-1	10.95	14.50
_____ Stay Cool Through Menopause	399-51818-5	9.95	12.95

Subtotal $ _____
Postage & handling* $ _____
Sales tax (CA, NJ, NY, PA, Canada) $ _____
Total amount due $ _____

Payable in U.S. funds (no cash orders accepted). $15.00 minimum for credit card orders.
*Postage & handling: $2.50 for 1 book, 75¢ for each additional book up to a maximum of $6.25.

Enclosed is my ☐ check ☐ money order
Please charge my ☐ Visa ☐ MasterCard ☐ American Express

Card # _____ Expiration date _____
Signature as on charge card _____
Name _____
Address _____
City _____ State _____ Zip _____

Please allow six weeks for delivery. Prices subject to change without notice.

Source key #48